An IVF Miracle
from Mahers

... including pregnancy stories of loss, reflection
and new beginnings (IVF and non IVF)

J Maher

Published by White Light Publishing House, 2020
Copyright © 2020 J Maher

This book is a recollection of true experiences over time. Some events may have been compressed, and some dialogue has been recreated.

National Library of Australia
Cataloguing-in-Publication data:
An IVF Miracle from Mahers/White Light Publishing
ISBN: (sc) 978-0-6450180-4-2
ISBN: (e) 978-0-6450180-6-6

CONTENTS

The picture below captures the height of my determination. The moment of triumph; when I obliviously, and contrary to medical procedure/advice, ripped down the blue sheet of the operating theatre after hearing my son for the first time. I could not see him. It did not matter what he looked like; but I needed to see him to believe he was there. It was at this moment I knew we'd made it. Thank you, my son, for giving me this magical moment in time.

My saving grace was optimism and hoping science would result in the fairy tale that IVF can be because I could not see the finish line. I now feel determined to help and inspire others so their flame of hope might also continue to burn.

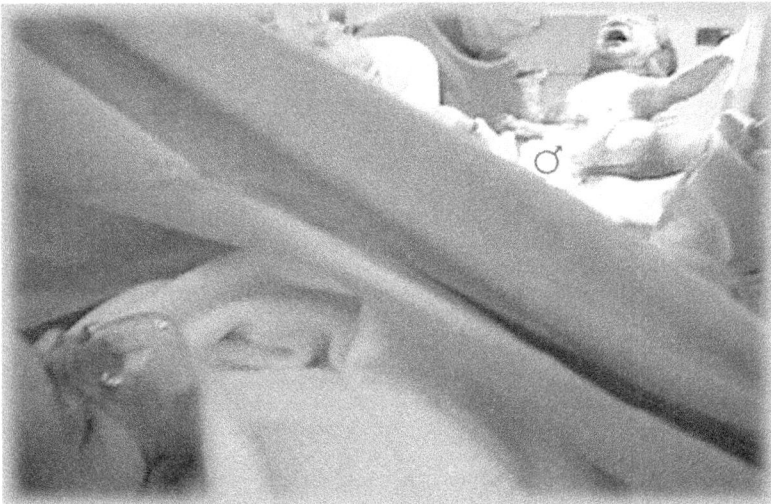

This book is dedicated to those who have a fire deep down in their soul to become a parent. With the resources available to you, give it all you can, and know you did your best.

Introduction

Infertility, and requiring medical assistance to achieve a pregnancy, is a predicament many people find themselves in. This can occur globally and it does not discriminate. It can affect both men and women and is a growing phenomenon. What causes a person to require medical intervention to achieve a pregnancy? In some cases, the answer may be found and can't be reversed, while others may achieve disheartening, unexpected or surprising outcomes.

In Vitro Fertilisation (IVF) is viewed as a common global-perceived fix to potentially achieve a pregnancy. The IVF patient numbers have increased, and in my non-medical opinion will continue to rise in years to come as health, medical, or biological reasons halt natural conception. And put bluntly, some instances may never be corrected, as I discovered.

If by sharing my journey to become a mother, I can inspire at least one person who wants to be a parent to try or try again, this book would have served one of two purposes for me. They are to inspire and encourage people, and to document this chapter in my life for my son. To these people I wish to inspire, I sincerely hope you achieve whatever it is your heart desires. I send you lots of love, strength and I hope the journey you travel is rewarding.

I read about a particular IVF case well into my journey and that was a defining moment for me. The lady had ten children and nine of those precious babies resulted in funerals. I was sad and the woman's determination connected to me. This was an example of a mother's heart in full force. Over here in my world, I felt I'd lost all hope. I felt defeated. This feeling was against the grain of who I am when I truly believe I must give my all. This story gave me the determination to find an extra layer of strength. I still think of this story after all these years. It deeply moved me and I will remain forever changed because of it.

The urge to become a mother is an overwhelming, primal and powerful force. It went deep for me. It was everything I ever imagined. When a woman is ready to have a child, it is what we desire the most in life. Just because I was a woman and possessed a heartrending desire to provide a beautiful child/children with all my love and comfort, the next step was never a guarantee I would get my desired result—a baby. I just knew I had to take that step. If I didn't, one thing was for sure, I would never become a mother and the thought of this left me feeling empty and fearful how I would ever feel content in life. This single thought alone forced me to dig deep when I was exhausted.

I felt a lot of responsibility on my shoulders, for the

family unit and my hopes and dreams, to successfully create and carry a baby, including significant worry when IVF didn't work. I accepted this responsibility with all the grace I could find and tried to remain humble when results determined I'd a chance to make it to the next step.

This journey tested my heart, soul, my belief in my ability to be mentally and physically strong, time after time. I lived outside my comfort zone and it was terribly sad and tormenting. I lived in emotional pain for many years. I mustered up strength daily, and it was heartbreaking. My eyes were filled with painful tears and my mummy-to-be heart was split in two through ten unsuccessful rounds of IVF. I just wanted to hold my baby.

I recall feeling at a loss and reminding myself that sometimes taking a leap of faith is the only mode of transportation. After the first two negative IVF results, I knew deep down, I may have to come to terms with the fact that IVF may not work for me. I tucked this thought away and tried to block it out (knowing, of course, it was still there) and I tried to power forward. I was reminded, attempt after attempt, that not having a biological child could really become my reality and this did not sit well within me at all.

I completely understand accepting what we have now and being grateful for the present time. Wishing for something in the future can be seen as saying 'now isn't enough' or hoping to make a dream come to life, as it was for me. I was so incredibly aware of valuing each moment in time because I knew you don't get that moment back to replay. I was grateful for everything I had and valued people who meant the world to me, I just wanted to become a mum.

I had an idea of the number of children I wanted to have in life, which was more than one child. Many people I have spoken to have the same idea or inkling, while others leave it to fate. Because of how difficult it was for me to become a mother; I knew I had to readjust my sails, which was a process of surrender and acceptance. I treated my pregnancy as the last in case it was, and it turned out to be this way. I knew I had to be present and not be lost in what my prior plans were.

Can we be happy with the numbers not going to plan? For me, that is a definite yes. I let my son guide me and he filled me with so much joy. I knew it was so important to be in the present, even though life sometimes doesn't fulfil your initial idea of what perfection is. My son was my story, and I never missed a minute of realising that this precious miracle growing safely inside me, was everything I needed to make me feel whole.

My heart really goes out to two groups of people.

• Those who have wanted to become a parent and despite trying to the best of their ability, they haven't been able to achieve this desire, whether that be naturally or with IVF treatment/assisted conception. Making the difficult choice to stop trying, or coming to terms with this decision would be one of the most heartbreaking moments a person who desperately wants a child can go through. Especially when the decision is taken out of your control.

- Those whose children have passed away before their parent hearts were ever ready/prepared for such a loss.

I'm so incredibly sorry and cannot imagine the pain associated with having to be in these situations. I wish these people and their families, lots of peace and love. I admire you for being so brave and courageous, through such helpless and uncertain moments. I wish you all the very best in life and hope you are okay.

While IVF can create a pregnancy with many successful deliveries, IVF does not guarantee a baby, a full term delivery or a live birth. My decision to undertake IVF was never guaranteed to result in a living baby for me, and while this possibility absolutely rattled me, it was a risk I was prepared to take. I knew very well, once IVF worked for me, that the outcome I wanted, which was a living healthy baby, was not promised and this made me incredibly nervous for the duration of my entire pregnancy.

Miscarriage, stillborn, premature birth and infant

loss have brought many tears to four special women in my life. With my deepest admiration and gratitude, I have permission to share their stories.

Thank you Renée, Rosalie, Kim and Kylie. We are new versions of ourselves with a story to share in the hope of bringing connection, comfort, unity, understanding and hope. We can assure you; you are not in this alone.

Rest in peace my 18-week stillborn nephew, Reggie (my sister Renée's IVF son), my nephew, David, who spent 117 days on earth (my sister-in-law Rosalie's son), six cherubs in heaven (my friend, Kim's babies) and three angels flying high (my friend Kylie's babies).

Renee also had one live birth, two miscarriages and the premature delivery of her daughter at 24.6 weeks (survived).

Rosalie went on to have two more children and dearly loves a third child she raised.

Kim experienced miscarriages, a baby born sleeping, premature birth (survived) and four live births. Kim was diagnosed with Polycystic Ovary Syndrome (PCOS), which is a complex hormonal condition with many problems, including reduced fertility.

Kylie went on to have four children and recently wrote a poem for her son Brayden's heavenly 21st birthday, which is chapter 30, 'Bedtime Story in Heaven.' Kylie hopes this poem connects to people around the world, who have suffered the loss of a child delivered sleeping.

I send a special acknowledgement to women from my mum and nan's generation who experienced the loss of a child. I hear stories of mothers never being shown their children who passed away during the childbirth process, as my Nan, Jessie, experienced with her son, Hector. Nan never got to see him, nor knew what happened to him. Some women, like Nan, were expected to just get on with it. These women must have suffered insurmountable grief trying to carry on with life. I witnessed firsthand how this is engrained within a person until they die.

I realise science, mental health support and medical procedures along with people's personal circumstances may result in more supportive scenarios nowadays.

I understand for some people, they may feel my medical journey is not that bad, compared to life-threatening injuries, serious illness or death, that they or others have suffered or witnessed. Every time I went to hospital, I sent a silent wish to anyone that was sick and hoped they would heal. I had incredibly sick people surrounding me in hospital and in my personal life. I was aware my scenario was, to a degree, a choice to start treatment again, and I never took this for granted. I know we are all different and our own story is extremely painful within. I send you lots of strength and encouragement and wish you the best possible outcome for your medical journey.

Each person has a different story and walk of life. Every person is entitled to decisions surrounding every baby they create, and my intention is not to make people who don't need IVF or medical assistance to conceive to feel guilty. I wouldn't wish the IVF torment (that I experienced) on anyone, so I'm genuinely happy for people who conceive naturally and don't need medical intervention. I breathe a sigh of relief for you.

Thank you to the pregnant ladies who were around me for being so thoughtful and caring, knowing my heart was broken because of my story. I wanted you to feel my genuine joy for you and your pregnancy news and wished you nothing but a healthy baby and safe delivery.

Thank you to the amazing men/partners who genuinely want to keep their families/partners at the first and foremost of their lives and treat them with dignity, commitment, loyalty and respect. Particularly as we, as women, manage the change occurring to our bodies and all the emotions associated with attempting/achieving a pregnancy and beyond. We feel a responsibility to try so incredibly hard to make your wishes come true to become a parent.

I'm not a medical professional (pregnancy or mental

health) and will never claim to be. These incredible human beings' study and train for years to help others. I'm forever grateful for their skill and kindness. My IVF Specialist and Obstetrician used their years of training and experience and I leaned on them to cope with the next step. They gave me hope and solid ground in between my tears. They had a plan and I agreed to try it. We tried eleven plans.

The medical information I refer to is my interpretation of what I researched.

IVF is ever evolving and as a result the plans I tried may have been superseded.

Please consult your medical team for an individual assessment.

To the support network of people who carry us when our wings have forgotten to fly, thank you for your guidance, care and encouragement.

I believe when we do our best and keep backing up through adversity; we inspire others, attract good things and weave miracles into the life of ourselves and others.

CHAPTER ONE

1000 needles, 1000 tears

Me: "I'm nervous. Can we take a photo please?" I wanted a photo of my baby the moment he was born. In preparation for my caesarean delivery, I'd just been given an epidural in my lower spine. I'd enough time to lie flat before it took effect. I was turning my head away from the male doctor, who was now conducting a finger prick blood test to check my sugar levels. I'd endured over one thousand needles over the years to this point, and I still couldn't look.

Male doctor: "4.3"

Me: "Oh good." I breathed a sigh of relief. I knew a higher reading would reflect my sugar levels from gestational diabetes were excessive, which could have been troublesome for my unborn baby.

Suction sound for ten seconds.

Male Obstetrician: "Sweetheart, I'm going to have to push on your tummy."

Male Doctor: "It will be a bit uncomfortable because you can't push so the doctor will do it for you."

Me: "Okay." My eyes open wide through amazement.

Male Obstetrician: "There we go, come on, bubby. There's a head, black hair." I look towards the video camera with an astonished look, raised eyebrows and a big surprised smile.

Me: "Can we get a photo please?"

Male Doctor: "There isn't much to see yet. He's hanging on with his toes."

Me: I laughed! I was rocking side to side on the bed as the obstetrician's continued the delivery.

Male Obstetrician: "Oh hello, here we are."

My baby hadn't been delivered; he'd just been seen for the first time by the doctors. I looked at the camera in amazement and the relief that overcame me was exhilarating. I couldn't see my baby behind the blue sheet, however the doctors confirmed they could. The delight in the male Obstetrician's voice indicated my baby was okay, and this is exactly what I needed to hear right now. I was so excited, and I felt a rush of happiness. My heart was racing and felt like it would beat out of my chest. The tears were ready to burst.

Me: *Dr Jyotica Ruba (my female obstetrician), I know you're concentrating over there on the other side of the sheet. Please, please, pleeeeeease deliver my baby safely because I can't lose him now. I trust you. Please speak to me and let me know my baby has made it.*

I was listening intently to every sound in the room, waiting for the cry of a baby to break through the doctors' conversations. This would be my first indicator my baby was alive.

Me: *As soon as you are out, my baby, please just cry so Mummy knows you are okay.*

I'd been hoping all my adult life the stars and planets would align and grace me with a precious child one day. I have always said in answer to this wish, I would accept whatever precious baby I am given, and the long-awaited moment was seconds away.

Machines continue to beep and I could hear suction noises. I'd cried out all the sad tears and only the happy tears remained. There were years' worth of tears I'd built up and reserved for this moment in time. They'd been parked away in a bubble of hope. They were ready to fall. The bubble was bursting. I couldn't stop the tears.

I didn't want to stop the tears. I could feel the lump in my throat. I felt the many years of being strong, against all odds, was about to reveal why I couldn't stop. I had a feeling of being able to release opposed to constantly holding on, that I had never felt before on this journey. My yearning mummy heart was about to be rewarded.

My time had come. This is it. The wait was almost over.

Dr Ruba: "Ohhhhhh… Happy Birthday. Ohhhhh… This is your little one!" She looked my way with happy and excited eyes behind her mask.

Me: *He's alive.*

The bubble exploded and the one thousandth tear burst out of my eyes and rolled down my cheek. Only this time, the flood of tears was from pure delight and happiness. The dream to become a mother was now a reality.

Me: "Hello my Jy. I'm your mummy and I love you with all my heart." And then I whispered to Jy, "Thank you."

CHAPTER TWO

Ready to be a mum. Now!

Mum was showing more with her third pregnancy and shared the wonderful news of delight to my brother Ian and I, that a new baby would soon join our family. Ian was thirteen and was three years older than me. Ian would share his room if the baby was a boy, and I would share my room if the baby was a girl. We were both excited at the thought of having a new brother or sister.

Mum was visiting her in-laws in Balmain, Sydney, Australia, two weeks before the baby was due to be born. She intended returning to our school at Killarney Vale, Central Coast New South Wales to collect Ian and I when the school bell rang at 3pm. Mum left Central Sydney on a train and was enjoying a conversation with her mother-in-law, Veronica. They were admiring the scenery along the majestic waterways which was below the train tracks. Mum felt a severe pain and realised her waters had just broken on the train at Hawkesbury River, which was halfway between Central and her destination at Gosford. This was truly an unexpected event and Mum tried to remain calm but felt helpless and held on to the train window ledge contemplating how she would have given birth on the train. No one carried mobile phones at that time. Veronica was looking around the train for people who could offer support should Mum give birth. Mum concentrated on her breathing and knew the baby was close to being born. I had the privilege of giving birth in a hospital. I can only imagine how Mum must have felt in this moment.

The train arrived at Gosford at 8.20am and Mum made her way off the train and walked onto the platform holding her stomach. There were no lifts at the station back then. Mum looked at the stairs as they escalated in height and thought, I don't know how I'm going to get up those steps. Mum said there was no other way. She knew she needed to get to hospital in a hurry, so she walked up the stairs holding firmly on to the handrail.

When Mum got to the top of the stairs, two ladies approached her and asked if this was her first pregnancy. Mum answered, "No, it's my third," and they asked Mum if she'd completed her breathing classes. Mum answered, "Yes," and a contraction started as Mum held on to the rail and concentrated on her breathing. When it passed, Mum had to walk down a set of stairs to get to the taxi rank. Veronica had gone ahead and hoped her decision to get a taxi and not to find a phone box to call an ambulance would be the fastest way to get to the hospital.

Veronica secured a taxi and opened the back door and by this time, Mum was on the last step making her way to the taxi. Mum was worried about possibly marking the seat of the taxi in case she gave birth on the way. Mum placed her tan coloured cardigan on the seat before she sat down as she greeted the taxi driver and asked him to please take her to the hospital as fast as he could. The taxi driver said he would do his best. On the way, there was a red light, and a truck stopped in front of them.

Mum said to the taxi driver, "Please hurry. Please get around the truck. I need to get to the hospital."

Mum said that light seemed to stay red for such a

long time.

When the taxi moved, and the hospital came in view, it was 8.40am. Mum said she felt for the first time in hours she may make it to hospital to give birth. She exhaled and her shoulders dropped in relief. Mum kept concentrating on her breathing and the taxi arrived in the emergency area. Veronica raced into the emergency section of the hospital and advised the staff Mum was about to give birth. The staff asked if Mum could walk or needed a wheelchair.

Veronica responded, "She needs a stretcher."

The staff arrived with a wheelchair and raced Mum into a treatment room before moving her to a bed. They removed her dress, which was wet from her water breaking on the train. Then they gave Mum a robe, examined her, and rushed her into a delivery suite. My beautiful baby sister entered the world at 9am, twenty minutes from when the taxi arrived at emergency under difficult and stressful circumstances. Well done, Mum!

I was so excited when Nan collected Ian and I from school and told us Mum had the baby. We weren't expecting Mum to have her baby for another two weeks so it was quite a shock. I would have loved another brother, but when Nan told Ian and I that Mum had delivered a baby girl, I jumped up and punched the air with delight. A new baby sister. That meant I would have a baby doll to share my bedroom with. I was so excited to meet my new little sister.

When Mum came home, I got to hold my beautiful sister. Renée had a full head of dark hair and beautiful skin. I was so in love with my new sister. I was watching her little face and listening to the noises she was making as she wriggled in my arms. I loved looking after my younger sister and would pretend Renée was my doll and look after her with so much affection. I made space in my wardrobe and drawers for Renée's tiny clothes and helped Mum feed, bath and change her nappy. I couldn't wait to get home from school to look after my baby sister.

Renée had a red velvet dress and a brooch with her name engraved on it. I asked Mum if I could dress Renée for her professional photos and Mum knew how much I doted over my sister and said I could. I was chuffed. I knew from this experience I really loved babies. I loved my sister so much and as I got older and cared for my sister, I knew when I grew up, I would have my own baby one day. I really believed this.

As Renée grew, I would put makeup on her, braid her hair and dress her up in my clothes. We would dance to Kylie Minogue's song "I should be so lucky" with our hairbrushes as microphones. Renée and I had a strong bond growing up, and I was part of Renée's firsts for almost everything she did. I was a proud big sister and as we got older, we would have sister days. One included a memorable day on Sydney Harbour.

As I became a mother, I appreciated Renée's birth and how frightened Mum must have been from a whole new perspective. Mum told me later she just made it to hospital and was worried how she would give birth on the train.

Mum told me she quietly reflected on her own mother's strength when she gave birth to her.

In 1950, Nan was nineteen years old and staying in hotel accommodation above a pub at 89 Goulburn Street, Sydney. Nan felt that she was going to give birth. She was unable to wake her husband. The lifts weren't working so Nan made her way down the spiral stairs and that is as far as she could go. Nan laid down on her tan coloured jacket and gave birth. Nan woke some time later in hospital and asked what happened. The nurse advised that she was lucky to be alive, as was her daughter, later named Cheryl.

I'm still amazed by the bravery and courage displayed by both my mum and nan on the day they gave birth to their children. I certainly had very strong and courageous women to look up to.

I assumed as I became an adult I would find the right situation and could have a child when I was ready, just like Mum did. I assumed this because I was a woman and my mum and my nan had children. That's about as much thought as I put into it.

I felt if I was to care for an animal or a child, I had to be settled within. In my twenties, I delayed rescuing a dog to call my own because I was a spontaneous person. If I decided to stay at a friend's house for a night or go for a week, I wanted to be able to go. I thought it was unfair to a dog to leave them at home when I wasn't there, which was also each time I went to work. So, I never got a dog through my single years. I would have loved one but wanted to be completely ready to give a dog a home that was the best I could give. My loyalty rang true with wanting to raise a child in the same loving and ready environment. It would have to be when I was ready for the commitment, because I would be responsible for my child's life.

I'd waited for the scenario where I envisaged it would be forever. That to me is a place to raise a child. I would have loved to have had children in my twenties, but it didn't unfold that way for me. I watched friends enter relationships that then set the path for children to follow. I hadn't chosen a career over a family, but fortunately I had a job I appreciated. I soon learned that life didn't go to plan or at times, our most heartfelt desires weren't met. I wouldn't have a child until I felt I was in a responsible and secure place. I had opportunities before but waited until I felt it was right for me. After all, it was my life I was driving. I needed to be content with decisions I was making and for a child, I considered that everything had to be 'right'. I wanted my child to have the best start I could give him or her.

When I was thirty-one, I transferred sites with my employer. I left my family I'd lived close to for most of my life, the comfort of my home and friends and moved to another state to be closer to my boyfriend. I thought the time was right and left the security of life as I knew it and made these changes to commence the next phase of my life. I can say I took a risk in every aspect of my life and I gave it my all.

It took a little time to adjust to everything as where I

lived and worked was new. Where I went to the doctor, dentist and hairdresser was also new. Everything I did was in a new environment and I allowed myself time to ease in by returning to my family on some weekends.

I was in a transition period and was missing the comforts of my old life, but also excited about what lay ahead. I knew this was probably a normal way to feel, and I soldiered on. I invested every aspect of me to build a solid family life that would hopefully endure the test of time.

I wanted the decision to agree to have a child to mean that I was ready in my heart and I knew once this feeling arrived it was time for me to bring a precious child into the world.

What I didn't know was that you don't really have that choice—we just think we do, and for some people, it turns out to be quite an easy process. For others, it's gut-wrenching. My head and heart were ready to be a mum. Now! But my body wasn't.

What a drawn out, isolating and painstakingly difficult experience this would turn out to be for me in the years that followed.

What lay ahead would forever change me.

CHAPTER THREE

The words a woman doesn't want to hear

I was settling into my new surroundings well. I was finding my way in my new job and making new friends. After a few months of negative pregnancy tests, I wondered if something was wrong and thought maybe it just takes a while.

I kept trying to conceive naturally. Life was good. I'd surrendered two levels of higher duties in my previous job to transfer to a new office, so I was focused on getting those two levels of income back. This was the income I was used to. I'd moved to where the head office of my organisation was and there were more opportunities available for advancing. I wasn't going to sit and wait for a promotion to find me. I started applying for positions I thought I would be great at. I successfully gained a promotion of one level, which thrilled me. It was still one level below what I was capable of, but I figured it was a start and I was on my way.

I was taking good care of myself. I was eating well, taking my pregnancy vitamins and drinking a lot of water. I'd waited so long to have a baby. I felt I needed to protect my body and look after it so I could be certain I wasn't hindering the conception process in any way.

I was looking around the house and chose a room of which I would decorate to become the nursery. I wondered if I would have a boy or girl first, or both. I was due for twins. They say twins skip a generation and my nan had twins, a boy and a girl. So I guess if this was true, maybe I would be next in line and the idea made me feel happy and lucky if it turned out this way for me. I wondered if this time next year, I would be a mum, something I wanted the pleasure of experiencing one day and sooner rather than later.

After filling the house to the rafters with furniture and setting up house and a lot of deliberation, I decided to sell up the three-bedroom townhouse. I'd move twenty minutes closer to my work and into a bigger house. I figured it would be best to make the move now before I had a child. I thought I would slightly increase my mortgage and it would be easier to get a bank loan without dependants or being on maternity leave, when I'd otherwise thought of moving.

I thought it would be a good move to have more

space in the house. I'd travel less to work (time and financial gain) and allow my child/children to travel less to the central area for work or university (should they choose to study). I decided it was a good move for two generations, so a 'For Sale' sign went up outside and the town house sold swiftly. I also sold my single life home near my family.

I found a lovely old house that needed a lot of work. The whole house was in 70s décor. The kitchen was timber and green, the dining and lounge room had really old wallpaper. There was an old timber panelled fireplace. The main wardrobe was old timber, and the bathroom was orange. It had a granny flat downstairs and I could see my child living down there as a teenager. It had a double garage that was under the main roof, which I thought was an absolute luxury. The house was old and needed so much work, but it was what I could afford and all the work didn't have to be done at once. Structurally it was sound and the rest, well I could sort that out in time and when I could afford it. The main concern was having a roof over my head for myself and my child/children when they arrived.

I didn't move out when some renovations were taking place to save money. I prepared dinner and peeled vegetables in the bathroom vanity and I remember having hot chips for lunch served on the washing machine which was being stored on the back verandah. I made do and was grateful for what I did have, not what I didn't have. It didn't matter to me how long it took to get the house in order as I was content and the rest was all material, which has always been secondary to me.

At the same time, I was writing job applications to advance back to the level I was familiar with from my previous position.

It had now been seven months since my first negative pregnancy test. I was previously aware it could take up to twelve months to fall pregnant naturally. I tried a different approach and monitored my ovulation with a product called 'Maybe Baby'. It was an ovulation tester which was easy to use, reusable and is a mini telescope which helps you identify your most fertile day and the ideal time to conceive. I placed some saliva on the small telescope lens and after a further few months of negative results, even with this form of monitoring, I decided it was time to investigate this matter further.

After trying to conceive for ten months, I visited my doctor in case I needed to see a specialist. I would have the extra two months having been booked in the system and waiting for a specialist appointment to arrive. Rather than seeing my doctor at twelve months and then waiting longer. They referred me to a specialist at ten months and had a three month wait for an appointment. I'm so glad I was thinking ahead and saving time.

I kept renovations going at home that I could afford

and knew it would be a slow process, but it didn't matter to me. I did what I could after I finished working full-time hours.

I deliberately invested my energy evenly into my home life, seeking promotions and having a baby. I knew I could juggle all these important matters as long as I looked after myself. I knew I would appreciate the commitment should they all work out at some point in the future.

I'm not afraid of rejection, but I am afraid of not trying what I know I am capable of or believe I can obtain through hard work and taking a chance or risk.

I applied for another promotion and was called in for an interview. I was nervous. I really wanted this level as it would put me back to the level I knew I was capable of. I prepared for the interview the night before and created a reference folder covering my research of the position and responses to anticipated questions.

I was a bundle of nerves walking into the interview room but said to myself that once I walked in the room; I was to leave my nerves at the door and get down to business. I felt I answered the questions well, but I guess you never can tell until they made the final decision. It seemed odd applying for a level I'd previously worked at, but it was my decision to surrender and move, so I needed to claw my way back.

I was not stressed in any way, nor felt I was taking on too much. I felt joy and happiness with all facets of my life. I was concerned why I wasn't falling pregnant but knew the specialist would help me unravel the mystery.

My specialist appointment was now two weeks away, and I still hadn't fallen pregnant after twelve months. I'm a big believer in seeking help from people who specialise in their fields of expertise and I was open to whatever the specialist may suggest I try. I wasn't in any physical pain so I figured there wasn't an immediate issue that needed to be addressed and I kept waiting for the appointment day to arrive.

I was pleased to finally be in the waiting area ready for my appointment. I felt like I may get some guidance or even a simple suggestion and maybe I might be pregnant soon after. The doctor took down all my statistics and suggested I have a test which was to insert dye into my fallopian tubes to check for any blockages. They booked me in for a few weeks' time and I felt pleased the investigations were under way. I went home and felt I was moving along with each matter important at that point in my life.

I subscribed to advertised positions within my organisation to be automatically advised when a position became available. I received a notification for two positions which I wasn't sure I could complete components of the jobs after reading the candidate kit. The application was due fourteen days later. I deliberated over the next few days about whether to apply. Sometimes the candidate kits are written with fancy words and make the job seem more difficult than it is. Other times it's as difficult as it sounds.

I decided I could explain to the interview panel I could learn any aspect of the position they'd question me about and I didn't have experience with. I also thought I would let the panel decide if I was unsuitable rather than me making that decision for them. If I didn't apply, they would never have known who I was and I wouldn't have had any chance at all and would have never known the tested outcome.

These positions were at a level I'd never occupied before. I decided that worst-case scenario, I would receive feedback on my rejected application or feedback from my interview for which I didn't get the job. I wrote the best application I could and felt happy when I submitted it. At least they would know I was interested.

I was absolutely floored when they contacted me and offered an interview for the harder one of the two positions. It was a real confidence boost, and I pictured my delight at being offered the position as I really wanted it. I dreamt for a little while and then I prepared like any other interview, listing my research of the position and my responses to anticipated questions. I was so nervous at the interview I could feel my throat drying up when I spoke. I answered twenty-two questions and I thought some answers weren't good enough. I tried to come up with an example of a similar position I was faced with, if not the exact scenario to the questions. I gave it my best and felt I became a little more relaxed as the interview progressed. I walked out of the interview room quite bowled over from nerves and had a quiet lunch to reflect on how I went. What I did know was even though I thought more about better answers I could have given; I'd done my best under pressure and I convinced myself I should now accept it's over and let be whatever may be.

On 01 April 2007, I went to hospital for the tube test and to say I was nervous was an understatement. I really don't like medical procedures. I walked into the room and robed up, and it made me shaky on the inside. As my heart was racing, I remember looking up to the roof as I lay down and I felt so anxious. I just wanted it to be over so I could wake up again and know they'd finished the procedure. I wanted to know the result of the test and boy; did it break my heart.

The specialist visited me once the results were available, which was almost straight away and said the words a woman doesn't want to hear. It was explained to me I had one blocked fallopian tube, and this was the reason I wasn't getting pregnant naturally. Well, at least I had an answer and breathed a sigh of relief. I asked how we fix it.

The specialist said, "Unfortunately, we can't fix it."

I expressed relief at having another tube and I thought maybe I could still fall pregnant with one tube. When I discussed this option with the specialist, she explained that based on where the blockage was in my scenario, that wouldn't be an option. I asked, "Does this mean I can't have children naturally... ever?"

The answer was, "Unfortunately, yes it does mean that."

She explained if one tube was blocked, it was most likely the other one was not working as well given the long history of unsuccessful attempts at falling pregnancy naturally.

I was not expecting or prepared for this outcome. It was as blunt as that. Boom. Cop that. I swallowed and in a worried tone, I said, "Pardon, can you please repeat what you just said?" I was in shock. I wanted another attempt to hear I'd made a mistake and heard what the specialist said incorrectly. I exhaled and dropped my head and my shoulders slouched. I was winded. In this moment, my hopes of having a child the way we all imagined came crashing down. I could have just sunk through the ground. I felt so weak.

The specialist explained I would need to undertake IVF to have a child. I had a ray of hope that there was a way, but I didn't even know what IVF was. I'd heard of one couple having twins through IVF, so that gave me hope it helps people become parents. I was desperate for whatever IVF was to help me get my own child. I was also shattered.

I never read stories through my early adult years about assisted conception. Mums had babies by natural conception. My mother and grandmother conceived naturally. It was a blunt reality my ability to have a child naturally would never happen, and it was a devastating and isolating time for me. If that's what hitting a wall felt like, I just rammed into it at full speed. The car ride home was a bit of a blur as I really couldn't process properly what happened.

I arrived home, stepped into a warm shower and cried. I cried it all out. I cried and cried and my head dropped and I concentrated on my breathing as I felt I'd nothing else but the basics to keep going. I promised myself I would look after myself and be gentle. I did not have a negative word or thought about myself. I did not think I was inadequate as a woman. I thought I would instead accept this card I was dealt and blaming myself for any reason wouldn't make this any easier, nor was it founded I could have caused the scenario I found myself in. I felt sad, but I am aware when we allow negative thoughts to come in that we are also listening. The specialist explained this happens to many women and the cause of the blocked tube may never be known.

I couldn't take any more that day. I decided to not

research IVF before bed as I needed to rest my mind and try to soothe my broken mummy heart. Life was about to take a sharp turn and I did not know what lay ahead of me. I just knew I needed to take a leap of faith with my thinking into the unknown and trust something good would happen. This is the exact mantra I kept believing. I chose a thought that was positive. Time would reveal all. What I did do was accept that today was gut-wrenching but tomorrow was a new day and somehow, I would get up and face it. I'm glad I did because there was a surprise waiting for me at work.

I woke the next day, and it felt like a bad dream and I hoped it was, but then I realised this was my new reality. I felt dented, like I'd taken a massive blow. I could have had a sick day from work to process the shock, but I knew I might sit around feeling sad and that wouldn't help me face anything. I knew I needed to get up and keep going. I arrived at work and opened my emails and to my surprise there was a promotion letter waiting for me. They'd emailed it during my sick day I'd taken the day before. I was feeling dented from the news that caught me unaware but I took this news as a blessing because the pay rise, however little it may be, would obviously go towards helping me fund IVF.

I felt like this was an omen to keep going. It felt like a lifeline. I couldn't believe I was so shattered about my medical news and was on such a high at the same time about my promotion. It was bittersweet. I'd never reached this level at work before. I hadn't even contemplated it. I'd reached the level I wanted to get back to and thought I may as well keep going.

I was so proud of myself for letting the panel decide if I was suitable. What a brilliant decision that turned out to be. They congratulated me at work as I'd really advanced a long way in a short period of time. While I was present and could hear people congratulating me, I was also disconnected and distracted.

I gave myself a moment to take in the promotion and be kind to myself, but soon after, while having lunch, I began researching IVF in more detail.

CHAPTER FOUR

IVF ... What is that?

I had lunch on my own this particular day as I wanted to solely focus on my thoughts about IVF. I read a lot of information. I'd heard about IVF and knew it helped people have babies, but that was the extent of my knowledge. The clinical, and not the passionate way of conceiving a child set in.

I read an article on the internet which said, "After your third attempt of IVF, you may need to accept that it isn't going to work for you." I felt vulnerable, scared, worried that I would never become a mum and hopeful I would.

I discovered IVF is the only chance for some people to have a biological child. This would be my only way of conceiving my own child. My infertility could be treated no other way. For less severe cases you can try fertility assistance and still try to conceive naturally. IVF became my light at the end of the tunnel that may produce a child/children. I was aware the word 'may' is not a guarantee, and I felt like solid ground was no longer under me. I did not know what would happen from here on in. What I did know was that I needed to try IVF, otherwise I would never know.

I discovered that IVF can be used for numerous reasons, including if you or your partner has:

1. ovulation concerns because of conditions like polycystic ovary syndrome
2. concerns with the fallopian tubes
3. if either person has been sterilised
4. endometriosis
5. low sperm or egg count
6. a wish to avoid passing on inherited genetic disorders to your children

If a person is at risk of passing on a serious genetic disorder to their children, are in same-sex relationships, have health concerns or serious medical diagnosis, or have not found their life partner, they chose or can be advised to freeze their own sperm or eggs, or investigate donor options for the same.

Healthy eggs or sperm can be frozen for future use in IVF treatments. For example, people who have cancer sometimes have their healthy eggs or sperm frozen, as chemotherapy and radiotherapy can affect your fertility. These eggs or sperm can be thawed later and used in IVF once the cancer treatment is over.

With this knowledge, I booked my IVF consultation appointment with my first Fertility Specialist who conducted the tubes test. I arrived armed with a list of questions about IVF. She explained the process. IVF is a procedure used to overcome a range of fertility issues. A hormone called Follicle Stimulating Hormone (FSH) which stimulates the production of eggs (oocytes) in the ovary is secreted from the pituitary gland in the brain. Injections of FSH will be administered daily by using an injection pen into the fatty tissue in the abdominal wall. FSH stimulates the development of follicle or follicles in the ovary which contain the developing eggs. The progress of the developing follicles is monitored by measuring the oestrogen hormone they produce using blood tests, and through watching them grow during ultrasound examination. They then join the egg and sperm outside the body in a specialised laboratory. Then they transfer the resulting embryo or embryos to the woman's uterus, where they grow into a baby.

I was provided with a pre-IVF checklist that I must complete prior to commencing IVF, which was: provide a current referral from my General Practitioner, conduct Hepatitis B, C, HIV, Rubella and blood group tests, obtain a pap smear, breast examination, diagnostic ultrasound, complete consent forms by the start of treatment and commence folic acid at the recommended dose of 500mcg daily.

They gave me an IVF plan which included one of a few possible cycles, and a shorter cycle called an Antagonist Cycle. This process would take four weeks from day one of my period until the pregnancy result. It would require me to attend the IVF clinic on day one and I would commence FSH stomach injections for 10-14 days. This would be in addition to the antagonist injections which would suppress the pituitary, thereby preventing premature release of the developing follicles. I was optimistic the plan would work for me and I thanked the specialist for her assistance and said I would see her again soon when she collected my eggs.

I walked out of this appointment feeling lost. I couldn't believe what I had to do. All the injections, the appointments, the waiting, the wonder and the cost. I thought, 'Why can't I just get pregnant naturally? Then I wouldn't have to do any of this and I felt angry and upset I was trapped in this new world.

I realised I needed to accept this card I'd been dealt and focus on this path now. I got my sadness out about not being able to fall pregnant naturally and trust me; it revisited me at times over the years and I definitely struggled with having to go through IVF. To handle repeat thoughts and feelings, I realise once you process something, it's an emotionally healthy option to not repeat the scenario and accept that your mind has already dealt with this. It wasn't to block it out; it was to acknowledge I'd been to this emotionally difficult place and series of thoughts before and came up with an outcome to power forward with. I tried so hard to think of a third person who cared about me giving me good advice and I tried to take my own advice. I felt I was in a daze and that the fog would clear, maybe after the first round of IVF, and this all would have been a bad dream. How wrong was I?

What I was grateful for was the advancement of science and technology, because if I was born generations ago, I would have heard I can't have children naturally and that would be it. I feel for the ladies from generations gone by where this diagnosis would have been delivered to them with no offering of any scientific assistance.

The pregnancy rates at the clinic I signed with were 60% chance of a pregnancy and 90% within 3 cycles. At this point, I was laying all my chances of being a mother on IVF, like so many other mothers have done before me. I was hoping for a miracle.

I read more of my information brochures about IVF and could not comprehend the enormity of it. I could not fathom that science could overtake a body like this. Knowing this was the way forward for me, I knew if I gave myself some time to process it, I would just do what they expected of me. I'd no choice. This is the survivor in me. I try to accept up front the things I can't change, then I allow myself to feel whatever I feel and work my way through it.

It saddened me I couldn't get pregnant naturally when I was absolutely stable, ready and certain this was the path I wanted to be on. I was still in shock from hearing this news a few weeks ago. This feeling of sadness for this loss and feeling grateful for the gift of science would be a sign of what lay ahead for me. The up and the down and the getting back up again. I'd hoped the solid ground I lost earlier would firm up again and the only way that would happen would be for me to fall pregnant.

CHAPTER FIVE

Mixed views about IVF.

There are many happy parents around the world from the marvel that is IVF. I have talked to many IVF patients. That makes me feel happy, because I know the pain of wanting to be a parent and not being able to through my unsuccessful IVF attempts. I have spoken to IVF patients who have tried to overcome their own obstacles and not getting the outcome they set out to achieve, which was to become a parent. They were grateful for IVF, knowing they had tried all their options.

I believe when people do their best, some people find closure to advance to a different phase. I found this comfort of knowing people did their best assisted them to continue to move forward beyond the IVF phase in their life. For other people in this situation, I feel the pain of IVF being unsuccessful is a sadness that may never leave them. The desire to have a child is a force that is just so strong.

There are also views expressed worldwide about IVF. I have read articles about people with not so pleasant opinions about IVF. Some people were bold enough to advise me in quite a confrontational manner I was interrupting with nature, and there are enough children in the world that needed to be adopted. At times, I really felt targeted for seeking some assistance. I believe we are all entitled to an opinion. If I may, here is mine.

As I write this book, there is another article in the news about IVF and the comment threads indicate people are 'mocking mother nature' and we live in a world of 'entitlement' and 'why not adopt'.

It would be like me asking why people use microwaves opposed to cooking on a stove, oven or fire like the world did before they invented microwaves. Why do people use microwaves? Because technology has advanced. Why do people drive modern cars? Because technology has advanced. Why do I have a child? Because science has advanced.

Regardless of an individual's beliefs or values, which I do respect all views and would appreciate the same, science is now available to help people have a child. We as individuals have the right to exercise that belief or value in the modern age. That may mean you choose not to try IVF. It may mean you do.

I respect we all have an opinion and view.

Walk a mile in the shoes of IVF torment and the dependency on science and you see how grateful and lifesaving this science is. I consider utilising science in this manner as the world does with cars, computer, phone, household appliances, and internet connections. Then I consider how delightful our experience has been with our new appliance from the modern age. This is how delightful IVF is.

We all have the right to choose a new gadget. Maybe you didn't have an internet connection twenty years ago, but you do now. Maybe our phone contract ended, and we got an upgraded phone on a new contract. A phone that has a bigger screen, stronger megapixel camera or even lots more features. Maybe we don't need it, but on some occasions, people buy it anyway, either straight away, as a new contract or saving for it. It's most of the time because that phone is on offer and has more features than the last time we purchased a phone or signed on to a contract. Granted, some people keep their old phones, but I think you understand my point. Some people can't go a day without using their phone. (They are so useful and keep us connected to the world.)

I yearned every day for my child. I guess some people feel they have a right to judge another. I'm okay with people who feel I intervened with nature or that I should have just accepted that I couldn't have a child naturally. That would be like me suggesting the majority of the world don't upgrade their phone next time the contract is due for renewal. The lines of people are out the door when brilliant technology is released. The big companies have conferences to sell their new product and people even sleep outside buildings to ensure they get the new product when the door opens, and good luck to them!

We, as IVF patients, are at times, frowned upon for using modern science to create a precious child. I'm shaking my head. This really hurts. The whole world has changed because of technology and modern science in my generation. I'm not that old, but I didn't go to school and use a computer. They came in the year after I finished school. It just doesn't make sense in the world we live in that offers a possible solution for infertility to not try. It would be remiss of me to not use the available options to help me become a mother, something I wanted to experience, knowing full well, there was no guarantee IVF would ever work. I'd accepted I may never be a mother and that IVF may not work. But why do some people think IVF patients have to stay with the options available decades ago? Because it's not traditional? Does it matter if people exercise all their options?

I feel for women who couldn't have children because the science of IVF wasn't available generations ago. I feel sad for the part inside them that wanted to be a mother, because that was me for ten rounds of IVF. I had a blocked fallopian tube, and I wasn't going to stand aside and do nothing about it when help was available. I'm a fighter and will exhaust all my options.

I turned to technology and science, and IVF eventually bypassed my problem. I never once thought I was entitled to have a child just because I was a woman (as some criticism suggests if you don't fall pregnancy naturally, then just accept it). I hoped I would bear a child, but who knows what lies ahead. I tried because that's how I am built. I value people's opinions and I take what I like and kindly leave the rest. As mentioned, I'm not scared of rejection, but I am scared of not trying. I needed to exhaust all available options to be satisfied I tried to the best of my ability.

I believe giving makes the world go around and the doctors and nurses in all medical fields, give so much to our community. They truly amaze me every day. I used to watch the Royal Prince Alfred Hospital show on television. I'd be astonished by the work of Doctor Chris O'Brien (Australian Head and Neck Surgeon) who passed away from a brain tumour, and Doctor Charlie Teo (Australian Neurosurgeon) achieved in their respective medical fields. Charlie saved and extended the life of a lady I knew. I think he is an inspiration in the medical field and I'm truly amazed by what this one man has achieved.

I'm also forever grateful to a highly regarded skin specialist for the care he has shown my family with his precision and vigilance. He made a call that saved a life. This was my mums and she would otherwise be weeks away from getting her affairs in order. Thank you so much, Doctor.

The scientific and medical world, including IVF, makes me feel grateful for such dedicated human beings who display commitment and passion to help others.

People make all the difference.

The newest phone - Wow!

Creating a child with assistance from science – amazing!

.

CHAPTER SIX

Round one - My fear of needles.

The cost of IVF cycles at various clinics in my home state were similar and the cheapest clinic was the first clinic I went to. I went with this clinic as I was satisfied with the service offered by the specialists for the price quoted. I rationalised this choice by thinking if I could get pregnant, why would I pay more than I have to? That would just be wasting money.

I completed my first appointment with my specialist and felt overwhelmed trying to process the IVF cycle and what I needed to do. All I needed to remember was to arrive at the clinic on day one of my menstrual cycle and I would brace myself with my fear of needles as I went along.

Two weeks after I found out I couldn't have children naturally, I commenced IVF. It was 14 April 2007 when I first walked through the doors into a brand new world. I hoped I would only have to complete one round of IVF. This would be one of two IVF clinics I would visit throughout this baby making process and I was nervous.

I reported to the reception desk and advised I was here for day one of my first cycle. A lady with a warm and friendly manner greeted me. I thought how important it was to have staff at the first point of contact who were soft and gentle. Their kindness made a huge difference because I felt like I was in a foreign country and wasn't familiar with any of the surroundings or procedures. I was lost. I knew I needed to pay for the full cycle upfront and made the transaction on my credit card. They explained I would receive a partial refund from Medicare. She asked me to take a seat and advised they'd call me for a blood test or the nurse would, based on who was available first. She encouraged me to help myself to tea or coffee. I looked around at the tea and coffee facilities but was too unsettled to sit and enjoy a cup of tea or my favourite, hot chocolate.

I sat in the waiting room and looked around at the people who were there. There were at least fifteen people waiting, and I wondered if they felt as nervous as I did. I wondered if they were here for their first cycle. I watched three more people walk through the door and form a queue at reception. One lady had a child about three years old with her and my heart sank. It also filled me with hope and I wondered what this lady's story was and if she had her first child by IVF. If she did, I wondered if I would be as lucky as she was. I wanted to hold my own baby. I wanted to watch my baby grow. I desperately wanted it now. I listened to the guidance the receptionist gave the lady with the child and realised that for the receptionist, it was a job and one she did with compassion and politeness. For me, it was my dream of having a child and this was huge for me.

I looked around and tried reading people's faces and body language. I was looking for nerves and uncertainty to see if they were feeling the way I was. I sat down and could feel a lady beside me who seemed tense. She kept shifting in her chair and was restless. We made eye contact, and I asked her if she was okay. It was bold of me to do so, but I felt I needed to offer some comfort to her as I could sense her uneasiness. The lady told me she was so nervous and was waiting to have a blood test today and would find out after lunch if she was pregnant. She seemed annoyed at the process and came across frustrated. She said people have children that don't want them, or don't want to fall pregnant and they do, or don't treat their children right. I could feel her predicament and having to go through what she had to and what I was about to do to become a mum.

I said I hoped she got the outcome she was hoping for and that she was brave to have come this far. I explained this was my first cycle, and I didn't really know what to expect. The lady told me it will be okay and I'll get through it and I never know that I could end up being pregnant first round. I was wary of saying anything that would reaffirm for her that her first round didn't work. She told me that if this round, which was round three, doesn't work she won't be coming back as she can't afford to. I felt sad. I took a deep breath because I was still feeling the sting of the amount of money I'd just paid for one round and I wished she would get the outcome she desired. I felt a little desperate for her as I thought she must be so brave to be facing the finishing line and not by choice, because of finances. I really wanted this round to work for her.

I picked up a home décor magazine off the coffee table to focus on the renovation project at home. I was looking for ideas for colour schemes. I liked earthy tones like chocolate browns with splashes of bold and shimmery colours. I looked around at the décor in the clinic and I liked the lighting and thought it created the right mood for such a nervous waiting area. I wondered how many people became parents from this process and how many would never.

I heard my name called and wished the lady sitting beside me all the best. I never saw her again, so I don't know if she became a mother from that round. I hope so. The lady who called me for the blood test took me into a room and I sat on the chair as she placed the strap over and tightened it around my arm. The lady felt my vein and I could have just passed out. I did not know how I would get through this blood test.

My fear of needles consumed me. I explained I really don't like needles, and the lady asked me to sit still and that it wouldn't hurt. I said I couldn't look and turned my face to the wall so far that I was looking over my right shoulder. I felt the needle break my skin and tried to think I was in a nice resort somewhere, anywhere but sitting in the chair with a needle in my arm. I concentrated on my breathing and I was thinking, 'Please hurry up, I can't do this,' and the needle was removed. Thank goodness, that was the hard part over. I wondered how I would get through the next needle but decided I needed to learn about the medication process and I tried to park my fear.

I returned to the waiting room to be called soon after by the nurse. I followed her into a different room and she introduced herself as Shiralee and said she would take care of me. Shiralee explained my specialist requested we change our previously discussed plan and try the Long Down Regulation Cycle, and provided me with my medication, which were the FSH for this particular plan and the injection pen to load vials of FSH into. She explained my IVF plan and showed me how to load and inject the needles into my stomach. I was to inject the FSH medication via needles at the same time every day and report to the clinic as advised by the phone calls received from the nurse who would read the blood results. She gave me my IVF plan and medication in a blue bag designed to keep the medication cool until I could place it in a fridge. Then she advised I would be contacted after 12 pm with the results and the next set of instructions.

I walked out of the clinic feeling proud of myself and I was certain I could commit to the plan and remember to take the needles on time. I reflected on this being a choice. This journey would be a choice and I was hoping luck would be with me and I would be pregnant after my first attempt. I felt like I wasn't alone when I counted at least twenty people waiting in the reception area as I left. All those people were hoping just like I was and I wondered how many would have their wish granted.

Some people have to do unpleasant medical procedures every day and this kept me grounded as I felt sorry for these people and admire them for being courageous. However, it didn't take away what I was really going through, which was huge for me. I was facing my biggest fear, and that was a needle and I could feel I wouldn't be able to dodge having needles to have a baby. I needed to somehow find the courage to face this overwhelming process. It would be like someone who has a fear of heights having to clean windows from the highest floor of a building every day. I knew I needed to face this fear head on otherwise I wouldn't have a chance of being a mum to my own child.

I broke the process up into chunks and thought I would do what I needed to do today and not worry too much about tomorrow. My mum also taught me to take one step a day at a time and to try not to project my thoughts too much. This approach helped me calm down a little.

I went to work and placed my medication bag in the fridge at work and made sure I wrote a note on my desk when I arrived to collect it before I left for the day. I received a phone call after lunch and was advised to continue the medication and return for another blood test in two days' time.

That evening, I loaded the injection pen with a vial of FSH and dialled the pen to the specified dose. I tore open an alcohol swab and wiped over a section of my stomach. I removed the cap from the needle and pinched some skin between my thumb and forefinger and couldn't believe what I was about to do. I pushed the needle in my stomach. I squirmed and wanted the liquid to inject more quickly so I could pull the needle out. I felt a slight sting and overreacted, I guess. It wasn't as bad as I'd braced myself for. One thing was for certain and that was, I couldn't believe what I was doing to have a baby. I felt weak but knew it was a lot of fear as the needle itself wasn't too bad. To this day, I still have a fear of needles. You would think it would have left me, but it hasn't. I have to remind myself of the moments during IVF when I thought the needles weren't too bad.

I returned for my next blood test a few days later and subsequently received the afternoon call to advise I was responding to the medication correctly and to return in a few more days for my first ultrasound. This scan would check the size and number of follicles that were growing because of the medication I was taking. I repeated having a morning blood test and ultrasound every 2-3 days over the next week and received afternoon calls advising the results.

It would become a real juggling act to get to the clinic and hope the queue wasn't too long and then arrive to work on time. Each time I would be delayed at the clinic meant I would have to make up the same time in the afternoon. This ensured I was paid as I needed to continue to meet not only my IVF commitments, but everyday life expenses.

The options when receiving the afternoon telephone call from the nurse were to continue as is with the medication, continue with adjusted medication or cancel the cycle because of overstimulation from the FSH. Fortunately, I could continue and was advised they'd book me in for the collection of my eggs. I was excited that everything went according to plan and I'd be having my eggs collected. They explained this process could be done with or without sedation. Given my needle fear, I decided to pay an extra $250 to be sedated as I'd used a lot of strength to get this far. I was counting every dollar and trying to be frugal with my living expenses outside of IVF to help ease myself through my fear. I'd literally felt my heart race each time a needle was before me. I felt I needed to help myself and minimise any extra stress and give myself a break.

I opted for the least stressful way. I thought maybe I could be carrying the egg which would become my baby and I didn't want to add any extra stress when I could eliminate it. This meant having another needle in my hand to sedate me, but it seemed the lesser of two fears opposed to laying on the bed awake as a needle was used to collect the eggs. I needed to be asleep; I couldn't face any more. So, they booked an anaesthetist for my upcoming egg collection.

To release the eggs from the follicles, I was required to have an injection, which was a mixture of liquid and powder referred to as a trigger injection. Surgery to collect my eggs from the follicles was scheduled at 1pm on 14 May 2007. The trigger injection was to be administered at home thirty-six hours before surgery. As a result, I went to bed two nights before surgery and was restless as I was concerned I may not wake or would sleep through. I set three alarms in the house to wake me at 12.55am, 13 May 2007. Through tired hazy eyes, I got up and found my medication and mixed the powder and liquid together and squeezed my stomach and injected the trigger at 1am and boy did it sting! This was the most unpleasant needle of them all. I made my way back to bed and fell asleep quickly.

I woke for what was Mother's Day 2007 and I hoped my little one was under creation. I wondered if I would wake the following year with a baby in my arms to be celebrating my first Mother's Day. I sure hoped so. I sat out the backyard in the sun and enjoyed some breakfast and wondered what would lay ahead for me in the next few weeks. Would I have enough eggs? That was my first wonder. I knew I'd done all I could. I'd enjoy a day off with no needles in my stomach because once I administered the trigger injection, I didn't need any more needles until egg collection.

I arrived at the hospital the following day with a bundle of nerves. I did not know what I was in for. I was bracing myself to face the needle in my hand to sedate me. I really was not looking forward to it, but I knew I needed to somehow stop worrying about needles all the time, but each time I knew it was close, my heart rate would increase. I found my way to the correct area of the hospital and was asked to change into the hospital robe and sit in the waiting area. Then I was called into theatre and asked to lie on the bed. I took a big deep breath and hoped with all I had that I would be okay getting the sedation needle and I'd wake to the news they'd retrieved some eggs from my follicles. I remember seeing the big light above me before drifting off to sleep.

When I woke, I was in a bed and was still sleepy. I wanted to speak, but I couldn't work out what was going on. I apparently was told I had four eggs, but I don't remember. I was too groggy to comprehend anything. I fell back to sleep. I woke again feeling more refreshed and asked how many eggs I have. It felt like an eternity for the nurse to answer me but it wasn't; it was two seconds. Time seemed frozen in this moment.

I was yearning for the answer to be a large number. What was difficult for me to deal with was the lady beside me had just been told she had no eggs removed. I was shattered for her because I knew full well if I'd received that news I would have broken down and cried. I had four eggs removed and felt ever so grateful, but I was terribly upset for the lady beside me. I didn't say anything to her as I felt it wasn't my place and she may not appreciate my compassion in that moment given I had four and she had none.

Once I was alert and functioning properly, I enjoyed some toast and appreciated food given as I needed to fast for the surgery. They explained I would receive a phone call tomorrow to advise if the eggs fertilised with the sperm and therefore, I would have an embryo/s. Phew. I took a deep breath. I still had a chance. I got dressed and walked outside the doors and felt the sun beaming and it warmed me up. I called my mother, sister and friends to let them know I had some eggs removed. I was a little surprised I only got four as I'd heard of people getting ten or more but was grateful after what I had just witnessed with the lady beside me.

I returned to work the following day and waited for the phone call. I was so nervous and anxious. What would happen to me if they called and said the embryos didn't fertilise? I didn't want to speculate and burn energy on what ifs. But the niggling feeling was definitely there. I tried to activate the positive side and just pushed out negative or pre-emptive thoughts and figured if I could do this for 80% of my thinking, then I could build up some positive momentum.

I kept my phone close by and waited patiently for the call. I noticed an unfamiliar number ringing on my phone and answered, hoping it would be the IVF clinic and it was. I was delighted to hear I had some embryos, however only two made it. I lost two overnight and was shocked they hadn't worked, but also relieved two made it. I really felt like I was in the hands of science now. They advised I call the clinic after noon the following day to check the progress of my two little embryos. That was it.

This would become a difficult waiting game. One hour felt like forever and I needed to somehow manage my way through another day. I tried to make it as easy as possible by not analysing every thought to the nth degree. I felt it was difficult to keep up this positive approach because the thoughts of worry could end up becoming reality. Maybe I wouldn't become a mum, ever. And maybe this first round won't work. Maybe my body won't ever create a child. Perhaps I won't respond to IVF and then what would I do? Maybe I would be positive and everything could come crashing down anyway. I remained focused on allowing the positive thoughts to rule my mind. I hoped these two embryos were a great sign and would lead me to my first child/children.

I was at work and trying hard to remain focused.

I booked meetings to ensure it would distract me and I'd focus on the important work I needed to complete. Once I finished work for the day, I grabbed a book to read as I needed to get lost in something. Biographies, autobiographies and memoirs are my favourite books and I chose a book from my personal collection. I don't recall the title but I remember getting lost in it and it was a great diversion.

I woke on day two since egg collection and was so nervous but glad I would have the outcome today. I had a solid breakfast to keep my energy levels up and waited for noon to come around so I could call the clinic. I dialled the number and my fingers trembled. I felt so excited and just wished that luck would be on my side today. They advised my two embryos were still growing strong and they'd need me at the clinic the following day for a day three transfer. I was so relieved. I knew any phone call could be a 50/50 chance, and I was so glad the odds fell my way today. I approached my manager and advised him I would need to take the following day as sick leave for surgery. He was an understanding and supportive man and wished me all the best. I needed people around me to understand, but also knew people couldn't possibly know the depth of what I was feeling and I didn't want to go into detail with my manager. I was happy he was easy going and supported me.

It was the day of the embryo transfer and I was still bracing myself I might receive a phone call saying the embryos didn't make it, so I was wishing the time away. I was also excited I'd made it to today. I just needed the embryos to hold on and once they were 'on board', I knew I had as good a chance as any other person who hadn't gone through IVF. The difference was I knew my eggs had fertilised, and this was comforting. A lady not going through IVF would have to wait until her pregnancy test day to discover this information. I was tense and nervous as I lay up on the bed for the embryo transfer. I'd never felt so exposed or vulnerable. I felt the stress in my body and hoped I could somehow talk myself into relaxing more as I didn't want to be the cause for the pregnancy not working because I was stressed.

They advised the embryo transfer was a success and I now could have a rest for the following eleven days and boy did this sound like good news to me. The thought of not having needles for over a week was bliss. They gave me a picture of the two implanted embryos and it amazed me. They looked like circles with lots of air bubbles inside them. I thought people conceiving naturally wouldn't get to see a picture of the embryo; they would see a positive pregnancy test result via a pregnancy testing kit or blood test. I walked out of the clinic feeling hopeful and proud of myself. I'd faced a lot over the last six weeks and I was thrilled to have made it as far as I possibly could. It was just a waiting game from now on.

I pondered about the house and work over the next

week or so, getting excited at the thought of becoming a mum. I was in the best position. The embryos were successfully implanted and I thought many people get pregnant first round and there was no reason I could think of that would stop me from having such luck.

As instructed, I attended the clinic for a blood test on the eleventh day. I was feeling more excited than worried. I think I convinced myself I was pregnant and all I needed was to have the blood test match the way I was feeling. Another needle, but if I could pretend I was on a beach under an umbrella relaxing, that would get me through. This is exactly what I thought as I sat in the chair getting blood taken. They told me they would call with the result after noon.

I felt like I was bubbling with excitement. I really thought I was pregnant. I had period symptoms, but they hadn't arrived and that was the strongest indicator I was still most likely to get a call saying I was pregnant. I attended a meeting as soon as I arrived at work and it went for one and a half hours. It seemed to take a large chunk of the morning and I was pleased when I walked out. I only had two more hours to wait, and I looked at my to-do list and tackled the hardest things on the list. I did this on purpose to divert my mind. This approach served two purposes. It ensured I was dealing with the hardest task on hand which required concentration so it diverted me from thinking about what was fast approaching and so I'd complete the difficult task. Then I had less difficult tasks left to do.

As noon approached, I kept my phone close to me, and then the phone rang. I thought I was about to be told I am pregnant. The nurse said hello and said unfortunately I'm not pregnant. I was deflated. I couldn't believe what I just heard. What happened? Surely they had the wrong information because I was certain I was pregnant. Looking back, it was hope I was hanging on to and I learned there and then, that hope sometimes doesn't eventuate into what you desire. I was so upset. I held back the tears and thanked the nurse. I asked what I do from here as I wanted to try again. She advised me to book in and see my specialist to discuss the results and the next plan. I asked how long it would be before I could start again. She replied it is normally a four to eight week wait for my body to recover and reset, dependent on the specialist's assessment of the round.

I got off the phone and went for a quick walk outside and cried under my sunglasses. Why didn't it work? Why? I did everything right? This is what it would feel like for a lady who tried to conceive naturally. She would have felt this way checking a pregnancy home test. I'd invested six weeks and called on inner strength and I was sad and lost. I wondered what happened since each step seemed to be as was expected. I remember looking in the mirror and I looked shattered. I wanted to be positive for the next attempt, but I didn't know how to process how I was feeling.

What I did was ring my specialist to book in for an appointment and I utilised my flex time at work and went home one hour earlier because I couldn't give work my all. I would have if not for the option of flex time and thought I will utilise it now because I need to go home. I went home and had an early night because I was tired and still upset.

I felt like I was falling into an unknown world and nothing I could do would stop it or save me.

CHAPTER SEVEN

What just happened to me?

I have deliberately explained the cycle in more detail in this chapter, after I went through one full cycle. My reason is because this is how it was for me. I needed to find my way through and learn as I went. It didn't matter what I read or heard before the cycle; it didn't make sense until I finished it. I am not medically trained; however, I have described what I could understand IVF to be. I discovered the following were steps I would become familiar with:

1. Ovarian Stimulation

Ovarian stimulation is the first medical step in an IVF cycle and it's a balancing act. By prescribing a carefully controlled dose of FSH and other hormones and monitoring their effects, bringing to maturity as many available follicles as possible, while also preventing them from ovulating prematurely. The follicles carry the woman's eggs, which are later fertilised with sperm to create an embryo (an unborn or unhatched offspring).

2.   Preventing premature ovulation

In this step, medication shuts down the communication between your brain and your ovaries so they don't release the eggs before the specialists can collect them.

3. Triggering ovulation

Ovulation is triggered by an injection thirty-six hours before egg collection surgery. Eggs are mature and can float free from about thirty-four hours after the trigger injection, allowing a four-hour window for egg retrieval.

4. Egg collection

The main surgical procedure in the IVF cycle is the egg collection, otherwise known as egg pickup, oocyte pickup, and sometimes egg harvesting. They carry out the procedure in an operating theatre.

5. Anaesthesia

There two options for pain management during the procedure. The first is a combination of sedation and local anaesthetic, the other is general anaesthesia.

6. Egg preparation

The Embryologist (the scientist who looks after your embryos in the laboratory) will also be in the theatre during your egg pick up. As they empty the follicles, they pass the collected fluid to the Embryologist. They use a powerful microscope to locate and extract the eggs. They then transfer the eggs to special plastic dish ready to be incubated.

7. How does IVF work?

What happens exactly when they fertilise your precious eggs with sperm and then look after your resulting embryos in the lab during those five or six days? In conventional IVF, about 50,000 to 100,000 washed sperm are left in a small plastic dish with the eggs. The sperm spend the next few hours getting through the layers of cumulus cells, and hopefully one sperm will successfully fertilise the egg. By the next day, some fifteen hours after introducing the sperm to the eggs, Embryologists will check to see if your eggs have fertilised by looking for pronuclei. In normal fertilisation, there should be two pronuclei, one from the sperm and one from the egg. Not all eggs will fertilise normally, which is common. My clinic considered it a good result if 80% of the eggs collected have two pronuclei on Day One.

8. Blastocyst culture

Growing the embryos in the lab a little longer before transferring them to the female lets the scientists determine which embryos have the highest development potential and increases success rates. The time between day three and day five in an embryo's life is critical because it's when an embryo switches genetic control from the female's genome to shared control between the female and male. This can be a point in the embryo's development where problems occur and waiting to transfer embryos beyond it is far more successful.

Once fertilisation has occurred, the embryo will divide and rapidly increase in cell numbers over the next few days. If the embryo is healthy and survives to Day Five - the blastocyst stage - it will contain between 75 and 100 cells. It is a three dimensional ball of outer cells (the trophectoderm) surrounding a fluid-filled cyst in which an inner group of cells, the inner cell mass can be seen. The trophectoderm or outer cells will then form the placenta, membranes and umbilical cord, while the inner cell mass will become the baby. An embryo needs two things to reach Day Five, which are enough energy and normal chromosomes.

9. Chromosomes

Embryos must also have the right genetic makeup to develop normally. In humans, genes are contained in 23 pairs of chromosomes. An incorrect number of chromosomes can lead to failure of an embryo to implant or to progress to a 'regular' birth.

10. Embryo transfer

The IVF procedure to transfer an embryo to your uterus is usually straightforward and painless: no more (or less) uncomfortable than having a pap smear. Many people think that the uterus looks like it does in most diagrams, with a cave-like interior in which transferred embryos can rattle around and even fall out. In reality, the endometrial cavity is a potential space. No matter what you do, it won't fall out!

11. Wait for pregnancy result

After fertility treatment, once you've completed all the stages of your cycle, there's nothing more to be done than wait for the time to pass before your results—whether you've fallen pregnant—are known. This downtime can be trying and stressful after you've reached so many milestones to this point in the cycle.

A pregnancy blood test can be conducted on the eleventh day following your egg collection. This can be the most nerve-racking time of the whole treatment cycle and it can feel like a lifetime. Many people will feel simultaneously elated (there's a new chance of pregnancy) and deflated (there is much less to do compared with before the egg retrieval. There is less information and, unless you have specific questions, there is much less contact with people at the clinic). Because you've been focusing on your body for the past four weeks (or more), you'll notice and analyse every twinge, symptom or sensation.

12. Unsuccessful Cycle

The disappointment of an unsuccessful cycle of assisted conception can be heartbreaking and at times can seem greater than your original experience of infertility. Your Fertility Specialist will review your cycle with you to assess why you did not get pregnant but the reality may be that nothing went wrong. Rather that the numbers just did not go your way.

13. Frozen Embryo Transfer

In a stimulated or fresh IVF cycle, it can create several embryos. Usually they implant a single embryo and freeze the rest. They store these embryos in a cryoprotectant solution at a temperature of -196 degree Celsius, which is the temperature of liquid nitrogen. They can keep embryos in this state almost indefinitely and successfully transfer into the woman's body months or years later.

14. Remaining cryopreserved embryos

After the required embryos have been utilised, an annual fee to store the embryos is charged. A decision needs to be made about what to do with embryos that remain in storage. The options are: save for a future cycle, thaw and dispose, donate to other people or to science. This decision can be extremely difficult for people to come to terms with.

15. What not to do during an IVF cycle

Amongst other requirements, the obvious were to limit alcohol and not to smoke, of which I did neither.

16. Side Effects

The side effects of the FSH would be Pre Menstrual type symptoms such as mood swings, irritability, bloating, sleep disturbances, headaches, tender breasts, tiredness, irritation or rash at the injection site.

CHAPTER EIGHT

Letter to the clinic

I decided to change IVF clinics and would remain with the second clinic for the next ten rounds. I changed because of research I'd conducted and discovered the second clinic had a better success rate. I knew the cost of IVF was slightly dearer at the second clinic, but I justified it based on the results and reputation the clinic had. They weren't much dearer than the cheaper clinic I went with first, who offered a wonderful service and clean clinic with informative and helpful staff. Most importantly, they'd created several pregnancies. I did not have a bad experience; I just had a feeling to change clinics and needed to follow that feeling.

This meant I would have a new Fertility Specialist who I found to be pleasant, experienced, knowledgeable and comforting. My specialist reviewed the paperwork from my first cycle and suggested a different approach for round two. My specialist recommended an Antagonist Cycle. The difference between my previous attempts on the Long Down Regulation Cycle would be the brand of the FSH, the timing of the injections and the commencement of secondary FSH. I waited the required time of four weeks which would allow my body to have two menstrual cycles. This would satisfy my specialist and allow my body to be able to recover to start again.

On day one of my second period, I arrived at the new IVF clinic and paid for the cycle in full. I felt I had a little more wisdom than the last time I walked through the doors to commence my first cycle. At least I knew what to expect this time, but it didn't make it any easier. It was still a new clinic and as a result, the process would be new this time around. I could feel the desperation of people wanting children in the air. My heartbeat elevated in the waiting room. There was a restless and uneasy feeling about people being forced into using science to fall pregnant. Obviously, there was no privacy and everyone knew why each of us were there.

I was determined for the minor setback of my first failed round to be something I would just steam roller over and try again. I was on a mission, although I was still terribly frightened for my name to be called because I knew that would be more needles. This seems like a strange thing to say, but the nurse asked me to breathe as she was taking my blood. I didn't realise I was holding my breath in anticipation of bracing for the needle in my arm. This blood test would show the base line of my hormone levels and allow the nurse who would call with the results after lunch to confirm the dose of hormones to inject. I set a reoccurring alarm clock twice a day at 7am and 7pm to administer my injections.

I repeated this process every few days over the next week and a half until I received a call which stopped me in my tracks. They advised me I needed to cancel this round because I had Ovarian Hyperstimulation Syndrome (OHSS). This meant my ovaries overreacted to the hormone medication and could, if the cycle continued, produce too many egg sacs (follicles) and further health issues for me. More severe cases of OHSS may require a stay in hospital. This is because OHSS can lead to potentially life-threatening complications such as extra fluid in your body, thrombosis, and problems with your kidneys, liver and lungs.

I was so annoyed and frustrated because I did not have any symptoms to make me feel unwell. Once this 'at risk' information was described to me, there was absolutely nothing I could do other than agree to cancel. I needed to accept what I couldn't change. I can't say I was prepared for this outcome; I'd done everything right so far and was upset my body was reacting in this way. They advised I needed to wait to have three periods this time around, which would be a two month wait before I could start again. I was advised to book an appointment with my specialist who would discuss the outcome of this round. I visited my specialist feeling a little disheartened. However, she gave me hope that there were more options she could try. She wrote an IVF plan and encouraged me to attend the IVF clinic after three menstrual cycles. I felt content after speaking to my specialist because I knew she wouldn't suggest an approach if she didn't think it wouldn't work. I had to place all my faith in her professional ability. I walked out of the clinic and took a big deep breath because, while I would have to wait eight weeks, I had my health, a plan and I could try again.

I was now ready for my third round of IVF in two different clinics under the care of my second specialist.

I tried to enjoy the next eight weeks as much as I could, but it was a terrible waiting game. I just wanted to be undertaking IVF so I had a chance to fall pregnant. Waiting around was difficult, especially as I'd just done that for four weeks only to face a cancelled cycle. It seemed like a waste of my biological time, but my hands were tied. I didn't do anything overly active as I felt a real sense to wrap myself in cotton wool so to speak. I continued to eat well and drink lots of water as I required this while I was going through IVF to help flush my body.

I attended the clinic on day one of my third cycle to the familiar feeling in the waiting area of yearning for a child. What was different was this time, it had been over eight weeks and I was so anxious to get started so

I could at least be in the running. I completed a full round of IVF, which took four weeks to do so. I waited in anticipation at work for the nurse to call me with my pregnancy result and it was negative. I just couldn't believe it.

I wrote the summary of round three in the last paragraph in ninety-two words. I did this in an attempt to show how short and sharp the sting of a negative result is. It was all over in one phone call and it felt as blunt as this paragraph ends.

Then the letdown process began. I started reflecting. I'd many moments of hope and pictured my baby in my arms many times during this round as I believed I would get pregnant by the third round based on the statistics I'd read.

I soon discovered the person on the other end of the line would become the bearer of good or bad news for any round of IVF if I made it that far. It felt so clinical.

The nurse said, "Unfortunately, the result is negative this time, Jodi. I'm sorry."

I said, "Oh, (silence), okay, thank you for letting me know."

I have to say I was shattered. I was desperately hoping for a positive result. I questioned myself. Did I just hear this correctly? I knew I had. I confirmed I had to wait four weeks before I could start again. I hung up the phone and went into a vacant meeting room and cried. A worry come over me that just wouldn't leave me and it honestly never did until the day I gave birth.

I called Mum from the meeting room and broke the news to her. I could hear in her voice that she was disappointed, but Mum never ever put pressure on me. Mum said she was proud of me and to look after myself and she will support whatever decision I make next. Mum was my rock. I said to Mum, "What if IVF never works Mum? What do I do then?"

Mum said, "Regardless of what happens, I will always be here to support you. Have a rest today, darling, try not to worry too much about tomorrow, you never know what lays ahead. If you want to try again, IVF may just work for you. That is your decision to make after you've had a good rest, my baby girl."

I said, "Okay, thanks Mum," because I knew she was right.

When Mum called me 'baby girl', her mummy heart was showing me all the compassion and love she could. Mum always said you never stop being a mother no matter how old your children are and what she meant was a mother feels her child's pain no matter how old they become. Somehow, through Mum's hurt, she rose above it like a protective lioness would for her cub. Mum didn't show her own worry and said the right words to soothe and carry me. There were one set of footprints and they were Mums. In a matter of minutes Mum helped to ease the sting of what was a devastating result for me. I took a deep breath and felt the calmness in Mum's response and let her words guide the next move I made.

I knew with pep talks like this from Mum that I would be okay, for now. I also knew it was terribly painful for Mum, so I was aware of not emotionally falling on her all the time as I also needed to protect her. After all, she was the woman who gave me life, something I was so desperately trying to give my child. I needed to protect my mum from carrying the extent of my pain, but at the same time, I didn't want to exclude her as I needed her and she needed me. I asked Mum to call my sister as I was becoming too upset to keep making these calls and also because I was at work.

I went back out to my desk and wondered if I would ever use the maternity leave my company offered. I wanted to be at home with my baby, but there was nothing else I could do. I needed to make a decision and my options were to stop, take time out, or commit to the next attempt. I knew the answer already. I wasn't done yet. I checked the calendar and planned the next four weeks of waiting in between periods and worked out if I would earn enough money to do another round.

My sister, Renée, sent me a message and said she'd heard from Mum and knew I couldn't talk. Renée said she was so sorry for the result and she loved me so much. She said to keep hoping and try again if I can and knowing me as she does, it meant I would back up again. Renée said she believed I can do this again.

I had a weekend away from the normal surroundings at home and enjoyed a relaxing boat ride on the lake with friends. It was nice to take in nature. The trees lined the riverbank, and the birds were singing. The sun was shining, and I felt sad about my IVF journey to date. It had a way of consuming my mind. I was on a forced break for my body to recover and it felt worse than undertaking a cycle, because it meant I couldn't start.

I was out in what I would normally consider a wonderful scene, but I just couldn't take it all in. I didn't want to wish time away, but I felt I was, because getting to the start line was an achievement in itself. I just felt so sad about why IVF hadn't worked to date and wondered how long I would have to keep doing this for. I had fourteen more days to wait, and I continued to force the good thoughts to the forefront of my mind and value what I had in my life, not what I didn't. This is where it felt like torment because I was grateful for everything I had; I just had a yearning I could not fulfil. It was hard to continue to park it not knowing if that would end up being forever.

I was trying to plan to catch up with my friend, Emma. My family and friends knew by now that IVF dictated everything I did. This included making plans to see them. I explained to Emma I'm confused with the dates on my IVF calendar and I would clarify these when I start IVF. I would then let her know when I can visit. I contacted Mum to let her know I may have to see her the week before or the week after Mother's Day and as always, Mum was easygoing and understanding. It was all dependent on day one of my period and in previous attempts, I felt like the stress of wanting them to come may have in fact delayed them. So, this time around, I tried to not focus on when they would come, which was difficult to do.

Each day I was waiting and waiting and waiting. I was overdue for my period and it wasn't because I was pregnant. I needed to keep waiting as I'd no control over this. They arrived three days overdue and after lunch, so I wasn't able to attend the clinic as required in the morning on day one of a period.

I made it to day one of round four and I sighed in relief that I could finally start. Maybe this round would be it. Maybe the phone call at the end of this round, hoping I would make it that far, would change my life.

I let my friends Emma and Peita know, in fact, all my support crew were waiting with me. I let them know I started the stomach injections in the morning and they lasted for twelve days. I would then have about five ultrasounds during this time and surgery is looking like 14 or 15 May, of which the latter is my sister's birthday. Maybe that was a good sign as my sister had been cheering me on each step of the way. She was my adorable little sister, who was all grown up now and I loved her to bits.

Emma said, "Wow, so it's all going ahead tomorrow. Are you excited or nervous? I know the answer to that already. It is really happening, Jodes. I am so excited for you and I can't wait for you to have some good news. I have started to put a few little things away for you, little things my boy didn't use and some magazines and books. Little things that kept me positive throughout my pregnancy."

I advised Emma that I started the injections on the day they commenced and said, "Nothing to it. I didn't even feel it, so even better. I am getting anxious and excited. I am transferring back to the job I was in before Christmas, which I loved, so I am happy." I can't believe I felt this way back then. I was petrified of needles but I found a place where I was having time out from the fear. Although, I soon realised this would be a rollercoaster of fear and strength.

Emma responded, "I am so excited for you, Jodes, I can't wait until June so we can find out the result. I have your little package here and keep adding things to it for your pregnancy."

I felt like I was always trying to fast forward time, because I wanted to finish the round to get the result.

Being a person who values time, making the most of the day and never wishing time away, I felt IVF forced me to think and feel differently. I was constantly challenging myself to be in the moment and enjoy life and this came naturally to me prior to this IVF world. It was hard because I was yearning for a child—my child that I may or may never meet.

After four failed IVF attempts, I was feeling the strain financially, but I just couldn't fathom why IVF was so expensive. I was aware of a cheaper clinic in Sydney but I couldn't coordinate holding down a full-time job in Canberra and travelling to and from Sydney.

I was emotional and full of the side effects of IVF, but I felt the need to provide feedback to the clinic about the cost. Looking back now, it was a bold move for me. When I wrote a letter to the clinic seeking an explanation for the cost, they justified it from their perspective. I am in no way disrespecting the IVF medical world and like any business; they set their costs based on their own assessment and are quite within their rights to do so. I just didn't know if I could meet the costs if the rounds kept failing. What else could I do but try to find a way? I wasn't ready to stop.

Emma said she had tears in her eyes reading the letter. She said she knew it was hard but didn't know it was that hard. She said she admired my strength.

Strength is one thing I thought I could control and kept trying to find the fighter in me. I often called on love to deal with adversity and now I was trying to find peace and hope via love, via being kind to myself, but I was so terribly sad.

CHAPTER NINE

The branch was starting to creak

I would call my Dad every morning at 7.30 to say hello. It was our daily ritual. I talked to Dad about how lost I felt. He was a simple man, and he was straight to the point in an inspiring way for me.

Dad said, "Darling, you just have to keep trying and beat it."

While I heard Dad, I felt I'd been doing that so far. I asked Dad if he would come and visit me soon and he said he would. A few days later Dad arrived, and I felt happy.

I planned a whole day out with Dad to show him some local sights of Canberra. We visited the National Museum which held Australian memorabilia and there were some interesting items. I noticed Dad looking at machinery equipment that would have been from his era. We both stopped awhile at the old car on display and the bubble-shaped caravan and my admiration for those old caravans is still with me today. I intend to make an outdoor setting in my backyard, out of a caravan that is no longer road worthy and restore it as a peaceful place to enjoy lunch. Dad loved the country and the mountains, so I took him up the big tower and he enjoyed the 360-degree view of the picturesque mountain view ranges Canberra offered. We also hired a canopy bike and rode side by side around the lake and Dad said his sore hip felt much freer after the ride, which was great.

I remember lying in bed one night when Dad was visiting, and I cried into my pillow. I never told Dad this. I did a lot of my crying in the shower or my pillow. I had so many things to be fortunate for in my life and believe me, I was. I had healthy parents, loving siblings and I was going okay but there was a massive gap in my life. I wanted a baby. I'd always envisaged myself with a family of two children. I don't know why it was two, but that is what I always felt and wanted. It had to be when I was ready and I was now ready for my baby in my arms.

As women, my mum, nan and Aunty Kathy were who I considered female pioneers in this family. They had hard times, but they never gave up. When I felt lost, which was often in the IVF world, I tried to see how they powered on and this gave me hope. Aunty

Kathy chose to have fur babies, opposed to having children. Mum and Nan had the children they yearned for. Maybe one day, it will work out for me too.

Having said that, I felt cracks appearing. I felt like the cracking noises before a branch snaps. I didn't want to break. By this, I meant, I didn't want to give in to the torment because if I stopped, one thing was for sure, my chances for having my own child would definitely be all over. It was up to me to keep going and delve into this unknown world I was tiptoeing through. I was treading carefully as I didn't want to fall too hard one way or another. I needed to stay upright and carry on.

It was a battle of my mind to keep going and hoping that luck would strike me at least for one of these rounds. But what if luck didn't come my way? Because after all, life doesn't go to plan as I was quickly learning. I tried to think about how I would get through life without a child of my own. I tried to test myself to see if that would be a place I could exist in, because there was no guarantee this road I was backing up and walking down again would bring the results I desired.

I couldn't fathom at this point a life without my own child. I needed to have my child, and I wasn't ready to give up. I knew that maybe I couldn't do this forever because either my eggs would decline in quality or numbers, which would mean I would be racing against the biological clock, or money would run out.

As long as I had my job, I could do my best to keep the money I was earning to pay towards IVF, but I couldn't stop the biological clock. I had no control over this and I knew if I stopped and still had viable eggs, I wouldn't know how I would handle the sadness in years to come, by stopping when I probably should have kept going.

I must continue to be in control of my own thoughts. I must stay strong. I must eat and drink properly. I must get adequate rest. I must turn up. Every day.

I supported the branch with positive thinking and walking one step in front of the other, day after day, week after week.

CHAPTER TEN

Dad falling asleep - forever

Dad learned his trade as a butcher as a young man in Ryde NSW and later moved to Phegans Bay, Woy Woy, Central Coast, NSW, when Ian and I were young. He changed jobs and travelled by train to Ryde every day to work in the Dunlop footwear factory. He would save fifty cents per week in his social fund for Ian and I to enjoy the Christmas parties with rides held on the company grounds. I held the title for the fastest runner in the girls running races, an accolade I was proud of at seven years old.

Dad often took Ian and I away camping in our younger years and taught us how to survive in the country. They were happy memories from my childhood and as a parent I can see my dad did everything he could to teach his children and show us love.

My dad was the type of man who spoke and you instantly felt comfortable. I often asked for his opinion as I knew that no matter what he said, I'd feel better after talking to him. Dad enjoyed playing cricket in his younger days. He loved country music and most of the time you would find him with a guitar strap over his shoulder and he'd be strumming along singing a song. Dad entered talent quests and I remember a dome-shaped hall at Ourimbah and I was waiting forever (it felt that way as a five-year-old) for Dad to get up on stage to sing and I fell asleep under a table and missed his performance. This hall was beside the shops I purchased tissues at on the day of Dad's funeral and I stared at the building, remembering Dad on stage.

Because of Dad's age and how fragile and unpredictable life is for us all, I really took time out to enjoy my parents for who they were as I became older. I appreciated the lives they had along the way to make things for us children as best as they could be.

When Dad turned eighty, I suggested we go on a Senior Citizens bus trip together. I wanted to stop my world for two days and step into Dad's world. I arranged for time off work and Dad and I boarded a bus for a memorable experience to the Southern Highlands. We visited the Sir Donald Bradman Cricket Museum in Bowral and being the cricket fan Dad was; he was mesmerised by the memorabilia. We sat on the cricket field nearby and imagined Bradman as a young boy learning cricket which would become his magnificent and high profile career. We boarded the bus again and played bingo. I won some towels and then realised I probably shouldn't have played and allowed the senior people to play at their pace but they insisted I keep the prize. Then we spent the evening at a magnificent country cottage and the breakfast the following day was fit for kings and queens. We boarded the bus to take in some local sights and then we stopped for a wonderful lunch at a local club, followed by an afternoon tea at a stunning lookout at Fitzroy Falls. The scenery was breathtaking.

I tried to get Dad away on mini weekend breaks as often as I could and Ian did too. On one occasion, we stayed at a caravan park at Tuross Heads, NSW. As the boat motor had recently blown up (in the middle of the lake), we couldn't take it out on this weekend trip. As a result, we hired a tinny boat from the caravan park. It still brings a smile to my face on this particular day we went out fishing. Dad had a bad hip that didn't co-operate when he needed it to, and he couldn't reach down to sit on the metal seats. I had an idea. I got the dining chair from the cabin we were staying in and placed it in the middle of the boat. I sat Dad on the chair and we laughed together as I rowed the boat out to the middle of the lake. Dad thought I was hilarious. I thought he was hilarious. He looked like he was the king of the lake and I'm sure the holiday guests thought it was a funny sight too. It really is one of my memorable moments with Dad.

Dad's neighbour was planning to drive to the town I lived in for a family event and knowing that I lived close by, they offered to take Dad with them. They suggested he could stay with me overnight while they attended their family function. That sounded perfect to me, so I met them when they arrived and took Dad back to my house to enjoy a lovely afternoon with him. He liked kangaroos and there was a country area close by where I knew there were plenty so I took him for a drive that afternoon. He enjoyed the animals and the scenery. As Dad's visit wasn't planned, I already had other family visiting and didn't have enough beds to sleep everyone, but I didn't let that stop me. I knew I'd work something out. I cooked a nice baked dinner for everyone and we told stories and had some laughs together. Dad wanted to give me one of his guitars and I asked him if he would sign it for me and he did. He wrote, 'To my darling Jodi, with love, Dad x.' He sang some songs for all the guests. I took a beautiful photo of Dad and me together and we were beaming with happiness.

I was at round five of IVF, and as I'd often spoke to Dad before about my heartache of it not working, I raised this again with him. He encouraged me to just keep going, and I explained I don't know if I can because I'm tired, worn out and I'm sad. He said to do the next step, that's all I had to think about. Simple and wise words, I thought. He wasn't being cold, uncaring or setting unreasonable expectations for me by saying the following, he was encouraging me as he knew how much I wanted a baby.

He said, "No Maher ever gives up."

I looked him in the eye and knew that was his way of dragging me out of the pain and showing his belief in me. I looked at the elderly man before me and realised he'd come this far by having this attitude. I felt a wave of calmness and responded after a big deep breath, "I won't give up Dad." I didn't know if money would stop me from trying again and again, but I made a promise to my dad there and then that I wouldn't give up.

I set up one of my camping stretcher beds at the end of my bed and planned to sleep there and give my bed to Dad, more so out of respect for my guest, my dad. He wouldn't be part of moving me from my own bed. He insisted on sleeping on the stretcher bed. I wasn't one to argue with Dad. I knew he would be warm and happy and feel like he was camping, which would have suited him. I woke during the night and heard him rolling over and sighed in relief that he was okay. Because of his age, I was getting worried he might just pass away. I cooked Dad some bacon and eggs for breakfast and ensured his bag was packed. I needed to take him back to the meeting point which was decided with his neighbours the afternoon before. When we arrived, I gave Dad a big cuddle and helped him into the back seat of the car. I put his seat belt on and said, "See you Dad, thanks for coming to visit me." I told Dad I would send him the beautiful picture I took of us the night before.

He said, "I look forward to receiving it, love."

I didn't know at the time, that would be the last photo I would take of Dad and I and it would also be the last time I would see him alive.

I was on a rare inexpensive holiday and it was 02 July 2008, and Dad called me and asked if I would like to call into his house and stay the night on the way home from my holiday. For the first time ever, I said to Dad that I won't stay if that's okay as he lived on the coast road and I wanted to drive home the inland route. He was fine with my decision, as he always was. I was due to leave on 04 July 2008 and commence the twelve-hour drive home.

On the morning of 03 July 2008, I decided, for no particular reason, to cut my holiday short by one day. After a 12-hour drive along the inland road, I arrived home in Canberra at 12.30am, 04 July 2008 and decided I would sleep in the following day because of the long drive. Dad and I lived four hours apart and normally talked every morning at 7.30am. I secretly made this arrangement to ensure nothing happened to Dad during the night. Dad would always wait for me to call before he had his morning cup of tea with his neighbour. I said to my friend at the time who would be awake early to please take the call from Dad as I would like to sleep in from the long drive home. He agreed.

The next morning around 8am, he came into my bedroom with a worried voice and said there had been a missed call from Dad's neighbour on my phone and I immediately shot up out of bed. I knew something was wrong because Dad's neighbour never called me. I called Dad's number, and no one answered. My heart sank. I was hoping Dad would answer when I tried again. He didn't. No one answered. Then my friend tried again and an unknown male answered the phone and he confirmed he was a policeman. I could see the look in his face while he was still on the phone, that my dad had gone. I started shaking my head and looking at him intently for any facial expression that would give away that Dad was still here. I couldn't see one. All I could see was sadness. I said, "No, no, no, not Dad, no, not my dad." He hung up the phone, and I said, "He's gone, hasn't he?" and the response was "Yes."

I hung my face in my hands and sobbed. My dear dad was gone. Through the sob of tears, when I could finally speak, I asked, "How?"

"He was found in his bed."

A tiny amount of relief came over me that if it was his time, at least I hoped he was warm and wasn't in pain.

I immediately grabbed my unpacked bags that landed on the lounge room floor seven and a half hours earlier and made the four-hour trip to see Dad who would be left where he was until I arrived. I called Mum to let her know Dad passed away and I could hear the pain in her falling tears. Mum was collecting money for the community at a local train station and said she would pack up and tell Ian. This made me cry. All my family were so sad and my brother was about to receive a knock on his door from Mum that would bring him to tears. I just wanted to cuddle Mum. The trip up that freeway is somewhat of a blur, although I remember a friend calling me and I answered and asked how she was. She was upset with her partner and was venting to me. I waited for her to finish speaking and she asked how I was and I told her I was doing a mad dash to see Dad as he'd passed away. She apologised for complaining during this terrible time for me and I said that it was okay, because there was no way she could have known. She offered her condolences and I felt her compassion.

When I arrived at Dad's unit, a policeman and my family were waiting for me (they'd arrived earlier as they lived closer). I said hello and had a cuddle and everyone had red eyes from crying. I excused myself and took a deep breath and walked up two stairs to Dad's front door knowing full well he wouldn't be sitting in the lounge chair about to get up and greet me. He would be dead in his bed. I walked through his lounge room and there were family photos hanging proudly on the wall. My mother, brother and sister were right behind me. I'd embroidered Dad a towel that said, 'Old Bastard'. It was just his sense of humour and it was hanging on the bathroom door. I made my way past the towel to his bedroom and my heart broke into two.

My eyes focused on my amazing father who laid peacefully asleep. Well, he looked that way to me. I wasn't in denial, but I wished I wasn't where I was right at that moment. I looked for signs of life. I needed to see for myself he really wasn't breathing. My heart was shattering into more pieces as my eyes confirmed Dad was really gone. There was no movement. I knew Dad was gone from the sequence of events during the morning, but I needed to see it for myself. I lost it. I sobbed. My body felt weak. Through the flood of tears in my eyes, I assessed Dad and couldn't see pain in his face but maybe he'd been gone awhile. I couldn't believe my eyes. I stared at Dad to ensure I wasn't in a dream and this was really happening. It was real.

I felt a force to be near him, as close as I could possibly be. There was no way I was not going to touch him. I was a little afraid as I hadn't seen Dad like this before. I laid beside him. I was absolutely broken. I was unsure if Dad would be warm or cold. I suspected cold. I held his hand and that first touch broke my world in two—the world I once knew and the world from this moment forward. I held Dad's hand, and he wasn't squeezing mine back. I sobbed. I cuddled him and kissed him on the forehead and his face was cold. Maybe he went to sleep for the last time in the early hours of the morning, or even the night before.

I felt under the blankets and there was still warmth. I became a bit frightened of how cold he was, but I continued to hold him. He was my dad, and I needed to hold on tight because there wouldn't be another chance for me to hold him like this. I looked at his face for a little while and tears kept bursting out of my eyes. My dear dad was gone. I felt like his spirit left and his body remained. There was no one in this body anymore. My chin was quivering from crying so much. I said thank you to Dad for all he did and gave to our family and said I loved him very much.

After a while, I walked out of the bedroom and looked around Dad's unit. It was a one-bedroom unit, and he was a simple and humble man. I tried so hard when Dad turned eighty to get him his own place as he didn't need to go into a nursing home and more so didn't want to. He was very independent and had planned to live for decades yet. Because of his age, he was placed on the priority list and offered this wonderful ground floor unit that was neat and tidy and suited Dad's need splendidly. Dad was so happy to have the toilet inside. Ian and I loaded the trailer up to move him from the place he was living in to this palace, as Dad called it.

The place felt empty, and I knew things would never be the same. I was shattered and was in a daze. I was grateful Dad passed in this beautiful unit and was in a warm bed. I looked around at the material items we acquire in life and to me; they don't matter when you are gone. Dad couldn't take any of this with him. I looked at the lace curtains which I hung for him two years prior when I arrived unannounced to clean up the flood in his unit from recent rain. I mopped up the floor and made sandbags and placed them outside his back door where the water came through. It was another reminder that material doesn't matter. The love we share, being kind and helpful and having good times with family and friends is what really, really matters. It was about all the times I stopped work, or plans I had, to ensure I could spend quality time with Dad. The memories we made. They were what matters and was vaguely sitting in the back of my mind mildly soothing me right now.

I looked for clues to tell me what time Dad passed away. I found a receipt in the kitchen for a purchase at the supermarket at 5pm the day before, so this confirmed Dad was up and about then. His shopping trolley was also out, so I assumed he'd taken himself to the shops, which is how he always shopped. This means he was active. After speaking to his neighbour, he confirmed he saw Dad the night before around 6.30pm.

The doctor arrived soon after and pronounced Dad dead from a heart attack. The funeral home arrived to take Dad away. I gave him a kiss again and told him I love him and always will and thanked him for being the best father he could be. I waited out the front with my family and watched Dad being wheeled in a body bag on a trolley from the door of his unit. Dad was leaving home for the last time. I watched the men place Dad in the back of a white van and they passed on their condolences and drove away. That was it. Dad would never come back here and I broke into a million pieces. I cried and cried and Mum cuddled me and cried with me. My feet felt heavy, and I was a weight on the earth at this moment. I felt like I would drop to the ground. My mum's cuddle was tight and felt like she was holding my weak body upright and I fell into her. I was trembling. I surrendered. My dad was gone.

I sat with my family out the front of Dad's unit for an hour or so and tried to come to terms that he wouldn't come back here. We all helped each other and shared some lovely stories about Dad. It was refreshing, and we ended up laughing as we reflected on good times. We helped each other to stand up and face the rest of the day. We'd earlier agreed on a funeral home at Ourimbah, which was a lovely big house on lots of land. Dad would have wanted this as he loved the open spaces. It was also on a road Dad often drove us kids down when we were young and off on one of our adventures with him. It's funny how you never know what the future holds. I drove past that funeral home for many years, not realising that would be where our family would hold a funeral service for Dad in years to come. I suddenly wanted to be a little girl again and drive down that road with Dad.

I was in the middle of round five of IVF and was

shattered to think Dad would never meet my child if IVF finally worked for me one day. I felt so sad. Fortunately, I remembered to pack my IVF medication prior to leaving home as I didn't expect to go home until the funeral passed. In the extreme events of the morning, I'd forgotten to have an injection in my stomach and just remembered I needed to do this as a matter of urgency. Otherwise my levels could be severely impacted to the point I may have to cancel this round. I quickly found my medication in the car and loaded the injection pen and administered the dose in my stomach. I hoped the few hours' delay wouldn't result in me having to cancel this cycle. I desperately wanted this cycle to work as Dad was with me at the beginning of it and this would be a connection to my baby if it was successful. I was clutching at straws to have a link to my Dad. I would have to wait until my next blood test, which was a few days away to know for certain what the impact was.

There'd been no warning. Six weeks prior, Dad was riding quad bikes with my brother Ian and sister-in-law Rosalie and I on a camping holiday. We'd all sat around a campfire singing songs and listening to Dad play his guitar. The day before he walked himself to the shops. We were in utter shock. I realise people live and then they die and my family wasn't exempt from the cycle of life and death. I just didn't want it to be real. It was so sudden and I wasn't ready for this, not that I ever would have been, but we were thrust into grieving and it was painful.

For a few years prior to Dad's death, I'd been donating a small amount of money from my fortnightly pay the Heart Foundation. I'd wanted to give some money, even though it wasn't much, it was what I could afford, to an organisation I considered extremely valuable in the community. It's ironic I was donating to this foundation and Dad died of a heart attack.

About two years before Dad passed away, he won $1,100 on lotto and added $50 per week from his pension to pay for his funeral. I tried to convince Dad I wanted him to spend his money while he was here and that my brother and I would take care of those matters at the time. He wouldn't agree with me and insisted on not being a financial burden for his children when he passed. Sometimes you just have to give in and this time was now for me. I respected Dad's wish.

In February 2008, when Dad was visiting me, I was teaching him how to use the Internet. He asked me what all this 'www' was about, referring to the World Wide Web internet pages he'd seen advertised. I explained what it was and looked up one of his favourite country music artists which was Hank Snow and he was flabbergasted at the amount of information I could find. He found a new appreciation at what the Internet was all about. I then looked at cars that were for sale and daydreamed about buying an old car, my mind set on only one brand.

I'd always wanted a vehicle matching the year of my birth and we stumbled across a bright yellow car which reminded me of the sunshine and I thought this one would just be fabulous to own. It was a 1973 Leyland Mini. I pictured Dad sitting beside me in this car and reliving his youth. I didn't have the funds to buy this car as they were committed to IVF and a baby was certainly more important than a want of mine and more so a material possession. I'd never asked Dad for money in my life. He was eighty-three years old. I knew Dad had some money in the bank, which he was using to save for his funeral. I had a feeling come over me and that was to ask Dad to borrow the money for the mini which was $2000. I felt like he may want to feel I need his help in that way. So, I asked Dad on the spot. When I asked him, he started crying.

"Of course you can borrow money from your dear old Dad."

I arranged with Dad that when my tax refund arrived at the end of July 08, I would pay him back. He was fine with this proposal but said, "If anything happens to me, please keep $1000 and give Ian $1000." I said that was a deal and that nothing would happen to him.

Dad asked me if he could have a drive of the mini and I explained it wasn't registered, but he certainly could when it was on the road again. One particular day, I left work on my flex time and therefore early and got some ice creams on the way home from the shop. I asked Dad to come and sit in the mini with me. His face lit up when I asked him.

Shaking his head in amazement, he said, "That's my girl. What a fantastic idea, let's go."

He walked to the garage with me. I figured if we couldn't take it for a spin; we needed to at least sit in it. We had a great photo taken together of us eating ice creams in the mini.

Dad died four weeks before I was due to repay the money to him. He never got to drive the mini as I'd committed my money to IVF and I couldn't afford to get it registered. But we got to sit it in together and what a precious moment that turned out to be. I captured that moment in a beautiful photo I cherish today. Once my tax refund arrived, I went to Ian's house, and he was shocked I was there to give him money. I explained the deal I'd made with Dad and needed to honour it, and it was emotional for him to be receiving Dad's money that he knew nothing about.

What troubled me for a while was if I'd taken Dad's offer when he called on 02 July 2008 to stay at his house when I went home, I would have called in and stayed the night of 03 July 2008. This meant I would have been in Dad's unit with him the night he passed away. This decision to go home from holidays one day earlier and not via Dad's was something that stung me for some time. I didn't want to indirectly torment myself by being upset at the decision I made. I believed if you make decisions that you feel are right then it was right for you at the time. Doing so wouldn't bring Dad back or change anything and Dad wouldn't want me to suffer. I talked myself into accepting that maybe I wasn't meant to be with Dad that night, even though I would have done anything to be with him when he passed away. It made me sad he died alone, but my comfort comes from knowing he was warm and hopefully he didn't feel any pain.

I clung to Mum even more so after Dad's death because I was afraid of losing her too. Mum helped Ian and I every step of the way and was a tower of strength in the time following Dad's death. I had a photo of Dad and I eating ice creams in the mini and wrote a note on it to say 'so long' to my dear father. I placed it in his coffin and kissed him goodbye. This really was the last time I'd see him in the flesh and I was absolutely devastated and didn't want the lid to be closed, but I knew I needed to let go.

I bought a brand new red jacket to wear to Dad's funeral as it was my favourite colour and made me feel better. I wrote the most beautiful eulogy and proudly stood before Dad's mahogany coffin. I took a deep breath and was focused on delivering the speech of my life. I told stories about a wonderful father and the room was packed. There were people standing as all the chairs were full. I didn't know some faces. I said to

Dad as I moved away that I love him and thank you for the memories. The song 'Moving On' by Hank Snow played at the end of the service and I pretended to play the air guitar in tribute to Dad's musical interests. I felt like smiling because the music made me feel happy. So, through the flood of tears, I had a big happy smile and felt the music as I'd done so many times before with Dad. The lady who led the service asked for everyone to give Dad three cheers and I smiled. He made many people happy, and we sent him off with a wonderful service. He would have been proud.

I walked out of the funeral home with swollen eyes and a heavy heart and nowhere near being ready or able to face the world without my Dad. I could see outside the cars were driving up the street and realised that life just goes on. I needed to somehow drive out of that carpark and push my life to go on. I owed it to Dad; I owed it to myself and to my family and friends that were still here with me and to the baby I hoped would come.

When Dad's funeral account was settled, there was $100 leftover in his bank account. Dad made Ian and I triple account holders a few months before he died. Maybe he knew, maybe he was setting things up for Ian and I to make it easier when he passed. I don't know how it worked out the way it did, but somehow the last pension Dad received before he died ensured he paid for the whole funeral with a little left over. Right down to the end, he was a man of his word. He said he would pay for his funeral and he did. Ian and I went into the bank together to advise them our dad had passed away and closed his account. They gave us the remaining money and we enjoyed a soft drink together from the $100. We were having a drink for Dad and clinked our glasses together and we said "cheers" for a magnificent father and reflected on our camping holidays with him as younger children.

I had that blood test and I was okay; the late injection didn't impact the cycle. So, while my dear dad had gone, I was hoping the link to him would make this IVF cycle work.

I returned to work after Dad passed away, but not back to normal. It would never be that way. It hit me with an unbelievable thud that rang loud and clear that my dear old dad had gone when I went back to work. I picked up the phone out of habit to make that 7.30am phone call to Dad and then I realised. I just had to, like everyone else who'd lost a loved one, somehow place one foot in front of the other and turn up to life again.

I continued to make choices that would have made Dad proud. I was now more determined than ever to create a life so I could look into the eyes of my child and know my dad's strength helped me create this beautiful soul. Since he'd passed away, his belief in me would keep pushing me to get up whenever I fell.

Dad's encouragement, strength and words would be

one reason I kept going with IVF.

"No Maher ever gives up."

CHAPTER ELEVEN

Round Five Result - 18

I woke to face another pregnancy result day and today was Wednesday. I hoped with all I had this would be the break I wanted and needed. I needed to get off this merry-go-round because I didn't know how much more I had in me to keep going. I wanted this round of IVF to work. I was desperate for this round to be a success. Like every other round, I did what they expected of me and to put it bluntly, I'd had a gutful of waiting and waiting. I was still grateful for IVF; I was just feeling frustrated, confused and excited.

I kept thinking of Dad and hoped if he'd left to make way for another, as they say, that this was an omen and a legacy Dad was leaving behind for me. I may just get my baby this round and I needed all the help I could find. The torment was stinging me. I wanted to burst. I wanted to escape the pain. I wanted to have a baby, so

I needed to keep going. I wanted to cry and cry I did. A waterfall for Dad, who I missed so much. A river for the child I wondered if I'd ever meet.

I'd previously heard of a couple undertaking five IVF rounds before they fell pregnant and thought that was a dedicated effort. That surprised me so much that they stuck at it for five whole rounds and I couldn't fathom how they just kept going. I couldn't process what they may have endured. Well, I was now in their shoes and hoped luck would be with me this time around, as it had for them. They had twins, a boy and a girl, and were deliriously happy.

I dreamed about receiving a call saying I was pregnant and pictured what the excitement may feel like. As I'd said all along, I will accept whatever I am given. It will be a miracle and a blessing rolled into one after what I had been through.

I went to the clinic on the way to work and the lady collecting my blood must have sensed I was a bit over it. She said she did eight rounds of IVF to get her child. I remember thinking there is no way I can keep going to eight rounds. How on earth did she do eight rounds? I didn't think I could keep getting up, but maybe I had to if she did. I thought I would be pregnant on this round and then I wouldn't have to worry about IVF anymore.

I'd spent a good part of the day communicating with my friend Emma. I emailed her at 11.40am and advised her that today was the day and I should know the pregnancy result by 3pm. Emma thought I expected the result in another two days and that she was so nervous. I'd stopped updating friends each step of the way because it had now been nearly one and a half years of a long journey for me. It just didn't make sense to update everyone at every stage. I could see my dear people were helpless, but they definitely offered me tremendous support. I realised they were struggling with this as much as I was. That didn't stop friends and family calling to check up on me; they were fantastic. I tried to minimise the weight for them to carry and internalised the deep torment and ache yet channel it as emotionally healthy as I could.

At 1.39pm, I wrote to Emma and told her I had a butterfly farm going on in my tummy and that I was extremely nervous this time. It was like every other time, but in the moment, it felt harder than the time before. I advised Emma that I would call her when I get the result. Emma responded at 1.41pm and said her heart was beating really fast now with excitement. She said either way it will be okay, but geez it would be great for it to work today.

At 1.47pm, I wrote, "That sure makes two of us. You're not wrong, I would love a break and to focus on the other side of a growing belly. How do I keep doing this, Emmie? The wait is torture."

Emma responded at 1.50pm and wrote, "You have

waited eight weeks through this round (actually a lot longer all up), so you only have one more hour to wait. All fingers, hairs, toes and nipples crossed!"

At 1.53pm, I wrote, "Yes, that is a good way to look at it. Thank you Em and yes, everything I have is crossed."

At 2.21pm, Emma wrote, "Can they drag it out any longer?"

At 2.52pm, I wrote to Emma with the outcome. "Got the call. They don't know. They said for a definite pregnancy my levels need to be fifty. For a negative result, it needs to be under two. I am at eighteen. It seems the embryo has taken but they can't predict what the outcome will be. I need to return in two days to see what the definite result is. I asked and was told some ladies have had a pregnancy from this result and some fizzled out. So, I continue to wait. Arrrrrrhhhhhhh."

Talk about dragging this out! Talk about tormenting me! I'd already had the build-up to the pregnancy call, and I did not see this one coming. I was expecting a yes or no, not an unsure.

I felt like the platform I was standing on and had been hanging on so tight to was wobbling even more. I often lived by a saying, "If you're not living on the edge, you're taking up too much space." Well, how true was this saying today! This result gave me my first glimmer of a pregnancy and I was thrilled that it could be a positive result. I was also guarded that it could be a negative result. I had, I thought, done my time and had enough negative results. My luck was due to change, and I'd be happy never to walk back into an IVF clinic again.

I had one foot in the positive world and sat there for a while thinking about it. I imagined so many things. There was a warmness about me and this time it wasn't me being positive and strong. This time there was a chance I was pregnant and until now, I could only imagine how this could feel. It felt magical. It felt real. I started daydreaming about being a mum. I don't know how things work when a loved one leaves, but if Dad had a say in this, maybe, just maybe, he'd been heard or orchestrated this result. After all, he was still on earth when I started this round.

Did Dad leave to make room for his grandchild to come? Was that the reason I could be pregnant this time?

I woke with one day to go to the second pregnancy result for this round and I felt troubled. I was feeling like I would break down if this result was negative. I hadn't had to wait two days like this before. I almost felt like I needed to bury that I'd completed IVF like I had to date and pretend I never even started. I felt like I needed to trick myself to be numb and that this wasn't happening. I don't know if I made things better or worse for myself, but I did whatever felt right with my gut feeling at the time. This was my guide, my leader, and when I couldn't decide, I just let my intuition take over and surrendered to anything else. To park away these troubles, I tried to enjoy the sunshine outside, the simple things. I tried to find some peace.

I felt like I would fall from a greater height if I wasn't pregnant, because this time around there was a real chance. I'd been shown that by the number 18. The pregnancy result call wasn't a no; it was a 'come back in two days' result. I was trying every way I could to remain neutral, but it was difficult.

I look back now and who I was back then, and I was such a tough woman. How did I do it? What other choice did I have than to do it? It was up to me to work out methods, theories and skills to cope while this pregnancy task ran parallel to my life outside of IVF. It was up to me to keep going, even when I was so unsure if this would ever work. And it was so tough I don't even feel like it was me who went through it all because I felt like I was a zombie.

Emma emailed me on Thursday at 8.36am and asked me how I was and mentioned she was thinking of me a lot last night. I responded at 9.23am and said I was fine and was feeling queasy for sure, but I'm being smart about how I handle the next twenty-four hours. Emma responded at 9.28am.

"I am nearly crying because I think you are pregnant. I don't want to get excited as you have been let down before, so I am open to the possibility that I am wrong."

I tried to switch off to the wait. I had over twenty-four hours until I would know the official outcome. It was an incredibly difficult thing to do time after time, but I knew I needed to curb this out-of-control feeling. I went to work and enjoyed my down time at home reading a book. I tried to force my mind out of my own zone and just be. I didn't want to just exist, but I wanted to rest my anxious mind.

I woke on Friday and took a deep breath as I faced the day. I messaged Emma and said today really is the day. I called by the clinic for my blood test, which I hoped would deliver the news I'd so eagerly wanted to hear—that I was pregnant. I pushed myself to focus and get to work so I could distract myself by being busy and achieving results at work. I was looking forward to the afternoon as I'd planned to make a three-hour drive to see my family after I finished work. I knew I'd arrive to them feeling happy or quite deflated. Each time my phone rang, my heart sank through anticipation.

I made it through work and was on my way to my family, which always meant a big warm hug from Mum and the thought of that made me smile. I was playing music in the car and was happy. I stopped for some food and while I was inside the building waiting to be served, my phone rang. I'd memorised the clinic's number, and they were calling me right now. I answered the phone and could tell by the nurse's voice I wasn't pregnant. As she spoke more, she confirmed it.

I felt my shoulders and my chest sink. I knew the drill from here. I thanked the nurse and said that all I can do is try again and to have a nice weekend. I hung up the phone and collected my food and walked out to the car and cried. It was a release. I was so sad. My potential link to Dad via a baby from this round of IVF was gone. My hopes were dashed. I sat in the car trying to eat my food but I was just staring into the sky.

Why didn't it work, why? Why did it take and read 18 and not keep going? Why, why, why? How do I get through this again? Will I get through this again? What do I do next? I took some time to sit and reflect and when I could concentrate; I continued to drive. I rang my family and friends on speaker phone and advised the news.

I'd discussed the negative result with Emma in more detail and asked her to please send me the link where she found the information about why the embryo doesn't stay attached. (Which she was researching while we were on the phone.)

Emma said, "Hi honey, it is technically a miscarriage. The embryo would have had to attach for hormone levels to start rising, which yours did. I hope that doesn't make it harder for you. It does confirm that the IVF worked, but nature wasn't on your side this time. I watched a show last night about a forty-three-year-old woman who was undergoing IVF. She had ten eggs, three didn't survive to fertilisation, three didn't survive the frozen cycle, and she had three miscarriages. She had one embryo left and had a beautiful baby girl. Hang in there, you are a Maher."

Had I tried to conceive naturally and without IVF assistance, I wouldn't have known the number 18. I would have just had a negative result. It was because they monitored each step. It made things harder because I knew my embryo attached and didn't hold on. I felt myself digging deep for courage in a different way.

I arrived at Mum's house with red, sad and tired eyes and fell into her arms as I told her the result. I could hear Mum's voice crack with sadness as she consoled me and said encouraging words. I heard the words, but I was defeated. Mum sat me on the lounge and made me a hot cup of Milo. I asked Mum what should I do next?

Mum said, "Enjoy your cuppa, love. You can't do anymore tonight. Get some rest. Tomorrow is a new day. You are fit and healthy and the next round was a new chance if that is what you want to do."

I told Mum I was so sad and what will I do if I can't

have my own baby.

Mum said, "Do all you can and take it one day at a time and try not to project too far ahead. Just look after yourself today and tomorrow and the next day."

I felt like falling apart, but somehow these words reached me. Mum had a knack of hitting the mark and soothing me. Mum thought of the future but could be right in the moment today. My mum had done it again. It was her simple approach that connected with me. I felt a fight in my tummy to carry on, but I had to get through this disappointment first. I hoped the dreaded feeling in my stomach would ease off over the next few days as the shock left my body.

Mum kissed me good night and tucked me into bed. The lights went out on a day that brought me my fifth negative pregnancy result.

CHAPTER TWELVE

If I stop, isn't it all over?

It seemed I was becoming more vulnerable each time IVF didn't work because the more options and IVF plans I tried, the less there were left that might work. I didn't know how many formulas we could try. I felt terribly cornered. This was an isolating place to be and nothing helped me. When I feel cornered, I come out with all the positive thinking I can muster. But this wasn't even working. I still wasn't pregnant. The worry of the failed rounds, and constant failed rounds at that, was compounding within me. I tried to somehow filter out the worry so I wouldn't hold on to it, but I didn't know how to keep doing this. I'd done so for so long and was just repeating techniques I used to push through the feelings of despair.

The pain of waiting and hoping was so difficult to manage. I wondered if I needed to see a counsellor at the IVF clinic, more so to talk about my heartache. I was feeling weaker from having to be so strong. I wasn't afraid to admit I was out on a limb here and if I'd professionally trained people available, my view was to make use of their skills. I would get all the feelings out. I'm open to people who specialise in their field to give me advice, because I'm the first to admit, I don't know everything. I tried my best to use all the techniques I'd learned so far to keep going, but I thought it might be beneficial to talk with the counsellor. I figured that was their job, and I was sure they'd seen plenty of people like me.

I knew I'd have to keep digging for strength no matter what the counsellor said. I knew the counsellor couldn't make me get a baby, but they maybe could help me find some peace in a different way or new coping methods. I felt isolated. I was exhausted mentally, physically and financially.

I made an appointment and shared my feelings and it was good to have someone who understood the difficulty. They suggested I learn techniques how to self soothe such as concentrating on my breathing. I have a deep inner ability to keep going, and I channelled all my worry into breathing techniques.

I started this IVF journey to get my own baby. When I was strong I would say, "If I stop it's all over and I'll never get my baby." This made me feel so vulnerable and weak because it was a reminder if I wasn't strong and kept being strong, I would have a whole new world to deal with. It meant not being a mum, and I wasn't ready for that. If I stopped, then what I tried to do so far would be for no result and I wanted a result. If I stopped it was certain I would never become a mother to my own child. So, I needed to do whatever they expected of me. I felt like I wasn't doing anything at 100% in my life. I was turning up, but I was really tired from juggling this IVF world. I was pushing myself at work. I was having broken sleep. I would practice techniques suggested by the counsellor and convinced myself again to be patient. Then sleep and do it again.

I still find it hard to describe the difficulty in how I got to round five. I was proud of myself, but I was so concerned that it may never work. I feel pain for people around me now who indicate they are undertaking IVF. I can see the angst in their face and I take a big deep breath.

I was aware of Deborah Knight, an Australian TV presenter, news presenter, radio host and journalist, who was struggling with conceiving through IVF. She had a public role, and I wondered how she just kept going, looked glamorous and turned up to work. I also wondered how she coordinated visiting the IVF clinic and arriving on air for a job dictated by strict schedules. I knew she achieved that feat, because I watched her on TV and was incredibly inspired by her ability to juggle it all.

The worry of becoming a mother seemed to consume me at home and at work. I was having trouble remaining focused because of the torment of unsuccessful IVF cycles. I watched Deborah conduct her job with grace and professionalism and I wondered how she mustered up the strength following unsuccessful IVF attempts and more so kept focused in such a public role.

Deborah had hair and make-up artists as part of her job as it is part of the uniform in a presenter's role. Make up makes people look different but it doesn't hide the pain in the chambers of our heart. I saw a really beautiful woman trying to juggle it all to become a mother. Every time I stepped out of my front door, I felt like I wore a mask to hide my pain. I imagined Deborah felt this way too. I wondered if Deborah felt like a shell deep down. An empty one at that. Just like I did. I had a quiet moment and sent her strength, courage and energy and hoped with all I had, that she, along with all the very sad Mummy's to be that I had come across, would get the outcome they were laying it all on the line for. We all just wanted our reality to be holding our baby.

No matter who we are, what we look like, what our employment is or isn't, if our home is spotless or to be cleaned, one thing is true. The heart of a woman from an IVF failed round still cracks in two the same. My heart snapped in half from sadness.

I had, at times, considered stopping IVF. I wanted to stop the torment involved with trying. I didn't want to stop having my own child. I only considered this because it was so hard to hang out on a limb and keep trying when there was no guarantee I would ever have my own child. It hadn't worked for me so far. I wondered whether it ever would.

I was taking a forced rest between round five and six for my body to recover. There was no reason why it hadn't worked for me up to this point. No medical reason, no explanation. Nothing. I felt like my chances at this stage were as good as winning lotto, which was slim. I don't like to talk about comparing feelings to money, but most people have bought, or know someone who has bought a lotto ticket. You buy it in the hope to win money. You picture how, with the winnings, you would buy a house, a car, help family and friends and donate to charity or even have a holiday. While you know the odds are slim, you buy a ticket anyway in the hope you may win some money.

I felt like I was buying tickets in raffles. Because it doesn't matter what you do after you've bought that ticket, it's out of your hands and you accept the outcome no matter what it is. If the ticket doesn't win, you know you still have the life you had before you bought the ticket. Well, I didn't want that life anymore; I wanted a life with my child in it. I wanted to win the prize. I was spending a lot of money buying 'raffle tickets.'

I now owned two credit cards to pay for IVF. One card would bear the cost of the full IVF cycle upfront. While I was waiting for a partial refund from Medicare on that card, I had the enforced wait of four weeks for my body to recover. I tried to pay as much of the gap that was owed on credit card one. At the commencement of the next round, I would have to pay the full payment on credit card two for the next attempt. I was juggling debt and scraping by to make ends meet. I wasn't defeated financially, but I was struggling and wondered how much longer I could stretch $1 into $5.

If I stopped, would that mean I was admitting defeat? I knew the moment I stopped, it was all over and I would never get my own child. The pressure this thought placed on me was hard to carry. I decided I needed to remain in the driver's seat and keep turning up. If I didn't, I was doomed and it definitely would be the end of an era I would never get back. There would never be a biological child if I stopped, and this did not sit well with me. This is how I knew I still had fight in me to carry on. I figured when I no longer thought this way, that was when I was well and truly defeated.

I was hopeful and excited about round six. I was also hanging out on a limb, throwing it all out there to see what would happen. I was feeling sore in the stomach from the injections. I was tender, and it was hard to find a spot that didn't hurt.

Fortunately, the hormone treatment produced

follicles, and I had some eggs, but they did not fertilise overnight. So, this means there was no eleven-day wait for a pregnancy test. It was all over now.

I remember thinking when round six failed, after eight weeks wait to start a different type of cycle, then the four weeks of the actual cycle, that even if I got a setback, at least I tried. Well, even this didn't sit well after everything I'd been through. I was praising myself for trying and I guess easing myself down from this whole IVF world. But it rang loud and clear once again, that if I stopped, I would never have my own child. This would be admitting defeat if I believed at least I tried.

What made me shudder with worry was the negative pregnancy test results. After the weeks invested, with no result, because that is what it was, became so excruciatingly difficult to deal with. I felt the ground could have just swallowed me again. I felt I was detaching from reality a little and what I mean is I felt no one could possibly understand the torment I was going through. My family and friends were absolutely amazing, but not one of them attempted what I'd experienced. I felt there were two of me. Jodi who was absolutely exhausted and tormented from disappointment and Jodi who had to respond to all my kind people with sadness, gratitude and a will to carry on. I just couldn't let them down. But I decided it was time to be real and be sad in front of them. Not all the time, but I needed to fall on safe people. This didn't take away from me that I was falling into an isolated hole and I couldn't relate to anyone I knew. It seemed no matter how I processed the pain or the constant negative results, there was a fire in my belly to get pregnant. So, I let my intuition guide me. I decided, that at least for a few more rounds, I was willing to back up again. I thought this approach may take away the pressure of the next rounding working, which I desperately wanted it to. I thought by being gentle with my thinking, that maybe, just maybe, the pressure might lift from me slightly. It might help me conceive this time around and I may not need to keep going back.

I'd put my car in to be serviced and as a result, I caught the bus to work this particular day. I noticed an elderly man waiting for the bus with an Akubra hat on his head, which is what my dad wore. Dad's hat was torn at the peak. He would say his hat was just like him, 'a bit worn out'. He had it for years and he wore it everywhere. This man had grey hair like my Dad did, and I sat and looked at him for a while. I really missed my dad that day and had a heavy feeling for him to come back to me for a while. If I could have him for five minutes again, I thought that would be fabulous. That night I dreamed Dad walked into my front door and walked over to me where I was sitting on the lounge and he cuddled me and then walked back out.

As I had done throughout this whole IVF journey, I tried to find the good in everything, anything that would give me courage to keep going through the agony I was suffering. I took this dream to be a sign to keep going. I made myself a promise there and then I would give this my best shot for as long as I could possibly keep going. I remember thinking to surrender and not put a timeframe on this, which in itself made me feel uncertain how things would turn out. But I was stretched to my capacity of wishing and hoping. I needed to accept this could go on for a long time yet. It was up to me how long I could keep trying and that was it. Accept it or not, so I accepted it.

Round seven was another twelve weeks of my life that was invested in IVF. A new IVF plan to try created by my specialist. They implanted two embryos for round seven as I was feeling isolated and needed to increase my chances. Implanting two embryos would give me a 20% chance of twins and this would be a blessing because I wanted one baby. Having two would be a pleasant and welcome surprise. One that I would cherish forever. Emma advised me if I have twins, I may feel sick quicker because my hormone levels double (or more than if you are having one bub).

Round seven just came and went. Just like that. Only this time, they advised during a blood test within days of the embryo implant, that there were pregnancy hormones and to remain aware these could be left over from the trigger injection prior to implant. They also advised my embryo I left for freezing didn't make it. It's the sting of these blunt outcomes that was hard for me. What I knew was I had all my eggs, which was two, in one basket—my tummy.

The wait to the next blood test was long. Being cornered to face my fear daily, choosing a different spot on my stomach to avoid the bruises there from previous needles. Making sure the zombie I'd become was fed and nourished. It was 3pm, and I'd been waiting since noon for the nurse to call me with a pregnancy result. I'd been previously advised the call would occur between noon and 4pm. I don't know how I didn't end up calling the clinic instead. I guess I was just hoping and couldn't face another sad phone call. I emailed my friend Peita and said to her that maybe they are calling all the pregnant ladies first. Unfortunately, the news wasn't good. My levels had dropped. My tears fell. Negative result again and again and again. I felt like falling to the ground and just laying down and taking the weight off me. I was tired from holding me up. I was sad. I was completely and utterly devastated. If there was a force stronger than me, I was wishing for help right about now. I felt that I was here on earth but I asked for help, from somewhere, from anywhere.

Each negative thought I had, I pictured it to be bowled over my head to the wicket keeper behind me. I needed to somehow take charge and to push the thought out of my mind. I questioned whether this was me escaping reality or being strong. I wondered how long I would have to do this for. I wondered if I would have to stop altogether.

Through all the positive thinking, I wished I could weave these thoughts into a magic rug that would whisk me away to a magical world with my baby. I was low at this point. I was down and I was out. I did not know what to do differently from all that I'd tried to this point. I was defeated. I was broken. I was lost. Money was drying up quickly. The odds were against me. I laid on my bed at home and just cried. I was being strong, I was backing up, but I lost it. I cried and cried. I'd completed seven rounds and done everything expected of me, and I still wasn't pregnant. I wanted to watch my stomach grow as my baby did. I was aching to be pregnant, but it just wasn't working out as I'd fought so hard for.

I told my friend Peita I want to give up, but I was dragging myself to keep going. I just couldn't take any more of the unknown. It's been going on for years now and it's driving me insane. Peita told me I was strong and she wouldn't have handled any of this like I have. She said she knows my dad would be proud of me and she knows deep down this is what I really want so she has to keep pushing me. She said she knows I will bounce back. Wow, I couldn't even see that in me. Thank goodness for my friends letting me lean on them constantly.

Emma said, "I can see why you are losing hope, Jodes. Your whole life is on hold until you have this sorted one way or another. I still have no doubt which way it will be, but I know that it would be hard to stay positive through this. The problem is only your tubes and not anywhere else, otherwise they would have found this in your tests. Like normal pregnancies, it has to be the right environment and with no defects in the embryo and that is something that cannot be controlled. The fact that your body was sore and tender and has been through stress of the surgery and not knowing what to expect, all plays a part. The eggs might have looked strong, but even the doctors can't tell at that stage if there is a genetic defect or not. You have every right to feel afraid. That is normal. Let yourself feel it. You still have a good chance of falling and tell yourself that you will have a baby, not might."

I didn't want to hear reason; I wanted a baby, but I knew Emma was right.

People would say to me it would happen in the right time. I agree with this. I agree things happen in the time they are meant to for you. This may mean we yearn for something and still may not get it, as the time might not be right for whatever reason. But gee, this was even getting difficult for me. Why was I forced to dig so deep time after time? Why? I kept myself grounded by thinking some people are dealt the cruellest health blows that lead to untimely deaths. The heartache the patient and families endure, and the medical staff witness in these circumstances is what is called 'not fair'. My scenario was a choice. Every month, I could try again. Every time I stepped into a hospital or clinic; I could walk out again. I felt awful for people in health predicaments where there is no way out and they have long-term painful processes to endure or even death. I tried to nurture my thoughts and keep them in perspective. I was healthy, had a job that would allow me to keep paying for IVF, even though it was getting harder and harder to financially manage. I had a great support network and a supportive employer. I decided while I had all this on my side, I only needed to think about today. I needed to continue to operate from the imaginary tank of fuel I had in my mind. This was for me to call on to keep me going when the going got tough. I was filling up on this particular day as I was feeling the compounded feeling of setbacks and wondered why this was happening to me.

I felt so exhausted that some days I wasn't putting as much effort into my appearance and while that's okay to have lazy style days; I noticed this world I was in was taking its toll. I looked in the mirror and my hair was a mess and my face looked exhausted. I don't have to look perfect every day, but I made a mantra of keeping the basics going, which was to eat and sleep well. I had to drink 2.4 litres a day through IVF to flush my system and found it so difficult in the beginning. I had times during the day where I would drink certain amounts so I could monitor my intake as I was reaching my daily target. I must say, I've never slept so good as when I drank that much water during the day. I'd also faced my umpteenth needle and braved my fear—again.

I extended my mantra and took a little more care

with my appearance and put in more effort. Even though I was drained, I knew it would make me feel better. So, I got up from crying my eyes out from sadness and walked to my wardrobe and put together an outfit for work the following day that would make me feel good about myself. It was a lovely shirt and skirt and the top was red which I knew would make me feel radiant. I straightened my hair and wore some light make up. I felt great going to work and knew it was up to me to keep the basics going for me. I was proud of myself for digging deep again in another way.

I read a story about a lady who had numerous pregnancies and numerous funerals until she finally got child through IVF. I read the story and wept. I was devastated for this lady and could not begin to understand what she'd gone through. Reading this story was a significant moment for me. I'm thankful this lady had the courage to put her hardship into writing. This was such a poignant story.

Each step I took from then on would be pushed along by this lady who never gave up and witnessed many of her own children's funerals. I imagined her somehow scrapping up courage to try again, and I was certain this is what I would keep doing.

Around the same time, Mum and I were visiting my grandmother in a nursing home. I stepped out to the car to get something as Mum remained with Nan. On the way back inside, there was an elderly man sitting by himself. I stopped and made a point of saying hello. He looked up at me and said, "Hello." I asked how he was going and he said he missed his daughter who lives in Sydney and doesn't visit him often. I felt sad, because I would have given anything to visit my dad. It was the second anniversary of his death that day. I sat and talked to the man for a while and he said I'd made his day. I don't think he realised he had in fact made my day and I let him know this. I thanked him for talking to me and advised him he'd made me feel happy. I felt a strength from this man who reminded me of my dad.

On top of reading the story about the lady who ended up with a wonderful child and talking to the elderly gentleman, I decided I needed to get back up and take this IVF world head on again. I remembered Dad's words.

"No Maher ever gives up."

That was it. I didn't know when the finish line would be crossed and whether it would be with or without my own child, but I was back and I ready to beat this. There was no way I was giving up. I had come too far. I didn't start this to stop. I found a renewed determination and I wouldn't let this beat me. I would do whatever they expected of me next, like I'd done so many times before. This was the Jodi I needed to come back, the Jodi who turned up to round one ready to take on whatever was thrown at her. I was still walking on unstable ground, but my mind kicked in a new level of determination.

I was feeling more vulnerable than ever, but the force of strength I knew I could muster from deep down was back and thank goodness. What I did know was there was a flame still burning inside me. I needed to find a log to throw on the fire. If I had to chop down a tree or a forest to get a log, I'd do it with my bare hands to get my baby. I found a renewed strength and look out, because here I come again.

I didn't feel there was a time when I said, "This is really going to work." I never had that guarantee from anyone or anything. Every round, every stage, every surgery, every needle, there was no guarantee, and this was extremely difficult. I was so scared IVF would never work for me and felt I needed to teach myself to live in hope. I knew how hard to date living with hope was because I didn't have the baby I desired. I pictured my child in all the stages of life. I was hoping today, and I'd wake tomorrow and hope again. I was wondering deep down if I was setting myself up for a fall, but that was negative so I pushed the thought out of my mind.

Through any hardship, I feel it sharpens your perspective and observation of other people and their behaviour. Something of which I am guilty of. I've asked people before, prior to my IVF battle, when they'd have children. Wow! How that question rips right through your heart when you are trying to and it's not working. I never realised before how assumption based this question is. It assumes people want to or can have children. I've asked the question freely, with the best of intentions, plenty of times and people who had only just met me have asked if I have any children. This is a conversation starting question and I understand that. But it was a tough question to answer for me, because I didn't know if I ever would have a child. If I answer and say I'm trying it seems too personal to divulge to a new person. I would just say, "No, I don't have any children." Phew, did this hurt. But I knew the answer was my reality and not how it had to end for me. I was shaking underneath from sheer worry that this may never work for me.

If I stop, isn't it all over? Yes, it would be. All over and every ounce of energy would have been for no return and that did not sit well with me at all.

CHAPTER THIRTEEN

Hurdles and Help

By this time, some people at work learned I was undertaking IVF. I didn't mind them knowing as I felt it was better to have a network of support than to do it on my own. I would just be selective about who I spoke to. They'd noted I'd being having some time off work, so I explained it was for a good cause and I was trying to have a baby through IVF. I didn't want to jeopardise my job and wanted to be honest. To make this happen, I needed understanding from my employer, and to hope for that in return, I needed to be honest, because I needed support. Which I got, thankfully.

A lady at work who'd done IVF came in to show everyone her new baby. She'd completed two rounds of IVF. This was excruciatingly difficult for me. I felt like I was using strength each time to deal with situations that tugged at my heart strings. It seemed each time I was tested; I needed to dig further and further to pass the test. I was devastated. I really was. I was pretty good at not showing my feelings as it would look like I was jealous when I wasn't. I was just sad and in pain. I didn't hold the baby as I didn't want to cry. I didn't want to show that level of myself at work.

Another lady who'd also completed IVF came in with her baby and wanted to meet up for a lunch break. When we sat down together she got the baby out of the pram and placed it in my arms and said, "Here, have a hold." It wasn't the right thing to do to me, even though her intentions were good. I didn't want to hold anyone else's baby. I wanted to hold my own. The lady didn't ask me, she just assumed that holding her baby would help me carry on. I held the beautiful baby and admired how adorably sweet she was, but the ground could have swallowed me. I felt so empty and desperate. It was the last thing I needed. I wondered how much longer it would be before I could hold my own baby, knowing that it may not even eventuate. I was dealing with something outside my control and my hopes weren't being met to date with my own baby. This lady asked me how IVF was going and I explained it hadn't worked to date and she said to just relax, stop stressing and take a holiday and it will work.

Really? This was another common statement people would make and to be honest, it drove me nuts. I'd heard this so many times before. I found it difficult to just do this because I needed money for IVF, not holidays. It appeared that she was assuming I was stressing. This could have been her observation of me, despite me not revealing a lot of my inner thoughts to her or her assumption when IVF doesn't work for people. I was relaxing to a point that other people don't have to find the skills to relax to. I just said, "Yes, I'm doing all those things." I didn't want to give depth all the time. I was tired and I felt like I was sounding like a broken record, so I gave positive and affirmative short answers.

I wanted to cry but worried I would turn into a blubbering mess and then would feel the need to explain myself as this lady, I assume, would have shown me compassion for crying. I held the tears in; I didn't want to have to deal with it. I wanted to go home and lay down and rest. But I went back to work as though nothing happened.

A lady at work made a comment to me and by this time, I could let negative comments just slide away from me. This lady said she didn't know why I was going to all the trouble for when there were plenty of children in the world to adopt. I said to her I agreed there are children to adopt. However, for my own heart at that point I had to do what I needed to do as I was driving my life and no one else's. I wasn't asking for anything abnormal. Women having their own children went on since time began. I asked her was she on the list to adopt a child and she said no, she'd already had her children. I asked why she didn't adopt one and she didn't answer me and then I think she realised her attitude was a double standard, one for her and one for others. I didn't want to justify why I wanted to follow through a dream of mine to a person who just made statements to me with no clue about what I was going through. I kept a brave face and figured she was only one person with an opinion and didn't invest too much energy on her. The alternative was to give her a big piece of my mind, but I decided that wasn't a wise way to invest my thoughts and energy.

Other people suggested adoption and I realised I needed to think about how I may manage this process. I couldn't seem to think about it deeply. It was like it was a second choice that I wasn't ready to process properly. In no way am I disrespecting children that would adore a loving home or the process, I was just numb and couldn't handle my own situation and how it was draining me. As a result, I knew it would be irresponsible of me to attempt anything I couldn't focus on. At this point, I couldn't cope with any more than what I was doing.

Adopting a child to me is something you must be extremely committed to. This is something I could have done. But I wasn't in the right frame of mind to go down this path at this point in time. I felt numb and there is no way I would create a relationship with a child unless I was ready and committed for life. It would not be fair to anyone involved. I knew adoption was a slow process. I'd heard it could take years because of my age (thirty-four). I didn't look into it at this stage as I wanted to exhaust all the options I had through IVF. It was a risk to not place my name on a list to commence the adoption process. I needed to follow my intuition, and that was to keep walking down the path I was with IVF. I was numb from my own experience and couldn't process adoption at this point.

A man at work told me I should have got into an arranged marriage when I was younger. He said if I did, I would already have had a child by now and could also have a deposit for a house (referring to the money I may have spent on IVF). I opened my eyes wide in shock of what he had just said to me and shook my head. I replied with a defensive tone, "Are you serious?" and he looked at me with an expression that confirmed he was. I didn't even respond. He'd no idea how I felt, he'd never asked and had no way of knowing how much IVF cost me to this point. I couldn't believe a person would say such a thing, and realised we all have different experiences and reasons and I excused myself.

I found it hard to field off some people's insensitive comments. Most of the time I could let it slide, but I also felt it was my job to stick up for myself to unreasonable people. I found while some people thought they were being helpful; at times it tested my patience at how ill-informed some of them were. I accepted people cared and had different ways of expressing it. I realise for some people, unless they experience something firsthand, they may or may not have an understanding and that's just the way it is. Other people obviously didn't think before they spoke. I continued to see the good and let any hurt by people's words just slide away. The most difficult circumstances to handle were when people made assumption based comments or condescending comments, opposed to asking. But it wasn't up to me to deal with anything more than I had to or could manage. I drew the line and put up a boundary when it was too sensitive or difficult for me. I wasn't rude, I just took care of myself because I knew I was dealing with extreme emotions daily while trying to hold down a job. I was already stretched emotionally and didn't have to take on anymore, nor did I want to when people were oblivious (and most not intentionally). I was also open to the fact that I was a walking IVF medicine cabinet and maybe I could have been a little too sensitive at times. I don't know. But I knew some things should not have been assumed about me, but I guess sometimes that is just people.

I wanted to remain social and open and not shut down, so I based all my decisions around this. I thought it would be disastrous for me if I gave up certain aspects of me or isolated myself because I was in pain. I was a bubbly person and knew I inspired people. I knew I was not built to retreat from my personality, but I was being challenged every day and it was hard to stay afloat sometimes.

My specialist wanted to do a biopsy on me to test the lining of my uterus because of the recurring number of unsuccessful attempts. I can't recall why this test was conducted but I do remember that the results did not discover anything unusual. I arranged a sick day from work and attended the hospital for surgery. I felt I was still stiff from fear of facing the needle in my hand as it frightens me. I pushed through the fear and did whatever they expected of me.

I experienced a particularly difficult time of the year around Mother's Day. There were now a few of them I'd pushed my way through. I focused on my mum and celebrated with her and realised if the planets align someday, I will get to celebrate with my child. I poured all my energy into making my mum feel special. I was teaching myself to enjoy with a passion the things I did have and while I had my mum, this is what Mother's Day was about for me. This wonderful lady who made many sacrifices in her life for her children. It was now her time to sit back and be rewarded.

It was very hard to switch off to the emotions and heartache. A good friend at work, Dana, knew this and was monitoring me and had been for years. I knew she would have done anything for me to tell her I was pregnant, but I just wasn't able to. During the time I was trying, Dana had taken maternity leave to have her beautiful child. Some women, and good luck to them, didn't understand what it was like to struggle to conceive. While Dana achieved her pregnancy with ease, she was so compassionate and supportive of my lost state. She was an angel placed in front of me at work.

She took such an interest and wanted to know

everything I was going through and as I felt so comfortable; I opened up to her and therefore have a friend at work who would be a soft place for me to fall when I felt down and out. This support was a real blessing for me, but I also didn't want all our conversations to be about how I was having difficulty falling pregnant. I wanted to enjoy people for who they were and not just for the support they could offer me. Dana would often call by and check up on me. Dana sat me down one day and spoke to me about adoption, and she was genuine about it. She explained that holding a child to call my own, regardless of the child being my own or adopted, she imagined would be a blessing for me and the child. I wasn't able to absorb adoption until this conversation. Dana had a way of making me feel at ease and helping me. I could see the relief in her face that I would at least think about it. Being a mother herself, she was kindly trying to help me get into a position to experience the joy she was. I needed to hear her and take on board what she was saying. It was the least I could do for a friend who was reaching out to me.

I was in the lift talking to a friend quietly about IVF and a lady spoke to me outside the lift and said she heard me say I was going through IVF. She mentioned she'd just started, and we sat down and had a chat. I'd had many unsuccessful rounds by this point. I don't know if that made her question what lie ahead for her if it doesn't work for her soon. I explained how I kept going and how I have to keep going. I could tell she was lost and was finding it difficult, just like I was. I was just a little further down the road than she was.

A lady at work asked if I'd completed a Cystic Fibrosis test at any stage of IVF. I didn't undertake this test because I'd already decided I didn't need to know. I wished for a child and would be grateful for just that. I would honour my word and accept the miracle I may be given.

A new lady joined our section, and her name was Cathy. I was responsible for teaching her the tasks in her new job. Cathy had two teenage sons and I could tell she was a lovely mum. We worked together for four years and during this time, I had several failed IVF attempts. Cathy nursed me through many rounds and gave me little gifts when I got the dreaded negative result phone call. It shattered me on the inside, but this gesture made me smile. Cathy was in tune with what may lay ahead for me and did little things at the right time to lift me up. The network of support at work was keeping me up, just.

Another friend from work, Amanda, who was also grateful for this world of IVF, had a difficult time conceiving her children for many years and we at times ran parallel with failed IVF results. When I first met Amanda, she was amid an IVF round and I could tell this woman had a lot going on. The common question I find with women when they get to know each other is talking about their house set up, including children or no children. Amanda had one child, a daughter, and had been trying for several years to expand her family. I explained I didn't have any children but was trying so hard to have my first. This friendship would develop over many IVF needles, frustration, tiredness, and later, one life changing phone call.

I completed one round without telling any of my support network, because I wanted to surprise them with a positive result. This was round eight, and it wasn't meant to be. I called on their support again for round nine. I needed people around that could push me, but I was also worried about being pushed into a false reality. What if this never works. How do I fall from such a great height? Knowing me, I would probably peacefully let myself slide down softly. If I had to, I would find a way, as I had throughout this painful and repetitive journey.

CHAPTER FOURTEEN

Hanging on by an egg

My friend Emma wanted to visit me. She was counting down the sleeps until we could see each other. There were eighteen to go, and we were both excited. I'd supported Emma through her pregnancy and when she arrived, Em was thirty-three weeks pregnant. I honestly was thrilled. I'm not a jealous person. I choose support and friendship over jealousy. Emma arrived, and I asked could I hold her stomach and wished her a safe delivery and said hello to her baby. I quietly wished upon a star that my turn would come. This wasn't about me; it was about Emma. This was extremely difficult for me to do. My heart was breaking for me, but I was ecstatic for my friend and I made sure she knew this.

I was facing my ninth round of IVF. This was an entirely different round because two embryos were available to freeze following round five. I made a strategic decision to leave these embryos in storage at the commencement of round six. The reason I chose to complete a fresh cycle and not use the embryos that were in storage then was because of my age. I wanted to leave younger embryos in storage in case I kept trying for years and wanted access to more youthful embryos at a later date if need be. I wanted to try as many fresh rounds as I could because each month I did they were becoming older and this increased my concern about how long I would keep producing viable eggs. The odds were slightly higher with a fresh stimulated cycle. It was now roughly one year between round five and round nine, so I decided to take those embryos that were one year younger than me out of storage.

I made this decision as I needed a rest while I wasn't resting. Let me explain. I needed a rest from stomach injections and I didn't need to have injections for a frozen cycle. It was only tablets and what a relief I felt this time around. I was still trying but having a rest if that makes sense. I could feel I was less stressed because of not needing to have injections every day. I hoped the removal of this stress would help me fall pregnant. There was a 70-90% chance the embryos would defrost successfully and the same odds for a pregnancy as the fresh (stimulated, injection) cycle which was about 35-40% chance of a baby. With my fear of needles still well and truly letting me know that it hadn't subsided, I was strongly encouraged to have acupuncture to assist me in falling pregnant. I don't know how I laid on the bed with needles sticking in my body for fifteen minutes. Everything I did was to increase my chance of having a baby.

I was so nervous the day before the embryo implant because I didn't know if my embryo would defrost. This was all new to me. All I knew was I could receive a call in the morning to say "the embryos didn't make it" otherwise if I didn't, I was to be at the clinic at 10.30am for the implant. I didn't receive that call. I explained to Mum that it would be silly of me to get lost in the expectation of being pregnant. I was trying to interpret what my body was doing and whether the pain was my period or a pregnancy. I couldn't tell as they have similar symptoms. They warned me my cycle wouldn't be normal as in timewise this time around, so I really couldn't even estimate when my period may arrive. I'd a feeling that it was negative and I am unsure if that was real or a forced feeling to help me get through the next pregnancy result. I'd lost sense of my intuition with detecting the result. It had been tricked and tested so many times I couldn't even rely on it anymore.

I said to Emma I feel sometimes I need to stop but somehow I keep getting back up again. I said I am proud of my determination and resilience and I don't know where it comes from, it must be the survivor in me. I asked if I was setting myself up for a bigger fall if this never works. Emma said she feels like bursting into tears regardless of the result and that she would prefer them to be tears of joy by a long shot.

"You are doing such a great job of handling this situation. You are strong and you should be so proud of yourself. You have managed to progress in all aspects of your life in such trying times. You will get through this, either way. We will all be here for you."

I got signs of my period and knew it was all over. I told Emma. She asked me to please go to the clinic in the morning and get a blood test and I said, "That would feel like a walk of shame." It was tormenting me enough; I didn't need a blood test to confirm it. Emma pushed me to get one as she said she wasn't convinced until it was 100% confirmed. I wrote myself notes to be strong if this result was negative. I left them on my desk at work. I was setting myself up for the next round already. I wanted a baby so much. I recall thinking I wished for my little eggie to 'go little eggie, go!' and was trying to stay upbeat. I also remembered that if bub was meant to be, it would be this time around. I was so anxious, yet still calm to receive the result, be that positive or negative, but I know what I was wishing for. I had the test and now I was waaaaaaaaaaaiiiiiiiiiiiittttttttttttiiiiinnnnnnnnnng.

I considered doing a home pregnancy test. I was caught in the pain of negative results and they continued to disappoint me. I waited out the process as I'd been through enough. I know the home test may have given me direction but it could have also confused me and I was tired and couldn't deal with anymore.

My period arrived when Emma was visiting, so that cycle was another crash from a great height. I was devastated. I asked Emma for help. I asked her to help me research if trying to unblock my tube would be effective. I told Emma I can't rely on one tube otherwise I would have/should have fallen pregnant prior to IVF. I said to Emma I didn't want to go into the detail of how I was feeling as I didn't want her feeling she needed to get me through all the time. Emma convinced me we were there for each other. Emma had to return home from her short stay with me to return to work.

I emailed Emma and said, "It's really starting to take its toll, the whole process. I'm not sure how many more negative tests I can handle. I cried myself to sleep last night. It's just becoming too much. I think the reality has hit that I cannot have children. I am relying on science solely and that is not working either. Maybe I need to sell the nursery furniture. I can only face the next attempt with no emotions, because I'm not sure how much more I can take. I feel I'm on the verge of cracking. I do not know how to bounce back and keep digging for strength. I have hoped through so many tests and I am over it. The only way I can handle it now is to give up or switch off and hand my body over and just let them do what they have to. I'm sick of pretending that I will fall pregnant. I have exhausted every option I have and I can't fall. I find I am a lot more negative over the past year than I have ever been, but I have also been under extreme pressure in this IVF world. I am giving up the will. If this doesn't work this time, I have no choice. I have to stop for the sake of not yearning anymore. Sorry to dump on you, Em."

Emma emailed and said, "Please don't give up hope. There is still so much hope. Your doctors have worked out what they need to do. You have a great chance for the next round because they know more about your body than they have before. Don't let your mind put you in a state of hopelessness. You need to stay positive and healthy for your body to be in optimum condition. I think you are stressed because you think this is your last chance. Don't put pressure on yourself. This isn't your fault and you don't need to feel guilty at all about it not working so far. The doctors know where your problem lies. Don't you dare think about selling the nursery, lady. I have more things here for your nursery. I won't let you give up. My intuition tells me to keep encouraging you. I am here to talk when you need to but I am sure you are feeling tired of talking so don't feel pressured to talk if you are tired. Rest my friend, lots of love Em."

I wasn't fishing for this chat from Em to prop me up. I was genuinely so lost and was reaching out and knew I could to Em. That was a dressing down I needed. Em's response made me realise she had faith in me at that moment in time, something I was struggling to keep finding. I guess I needed to keep going because I couldn't let people down, most of all not my baby. They were after all on this experience with me and how could I not try another round not only for myself but for my support network? I just didn't know how to, but I remembered I only had to take one step at a time. Right now, Em was carrying me emotionally. I'd surrendered to her and let her tell me what to do next because I was lost.

I sat on my favourite chair in the backyard under the pear tree. I held my head in my hands in despair. I decided my energy must remain sharp and strong if I were to keep going. At this time Renée called. She said she has a good feeling and that if I want something to ask for it and you will receive. I know she was trying to help me. I turned to the sky and politely asked to be graced with my Miracle from Mahers.

Come my way, my miracle baby.

Renée was ten years younger than me and wasn't in the phase of having babies at the time, but she was so supportive. One day she said she read an article about thinking of IVF as an illness. That when you are sick, you treat the sickness with home remedies or medication. She said some antibiotics clear the sickness and some don't. What I perceived it to be for IVF was, if one round doesn't work, see what plan you come up with the doctor for the next round. This information stayed with me and helped me separate one attempt to the next. I liked how simple this sounded. I needed to be pulled out of the depths of despair and with this kind of support I knew I would remain grounded. I took all the good advice I could find and kept topping up my tank of strength with it.

Leading up to this point, Renée would take me to

the movies and spend genuine quality time with me. It was a continuation of our sister days when we were younger. I remembered feeling so delighted when I heard Mum had a girl and my beautiful sister was all grown up supporting me. It was my job to look after my little sister, but here she was taking the lead because she knew I was struggling. I told her I was worried it may never take because they can't say why it didn't work this time, so how do they know how to fix it for the next round. She responded, "Each time it doesn't work, the doctors have something else to consider trying and to see this in a positive way." I could see the reason and trusted my sister because I was tired of analysing.

I sat outside until the sun fell away behind the mountains and decided I would take a big deep breath and try IVF again.

CHAPTER FIFTEEN

Ten and Tubes

I tried another round. It was another failed attempt. Yes, there were now ten unsuccessful rounds. I was now clutching at anything I could find to stop the negative results. I did not know what else to do. I felt weak. I felt beat. I felt defeated.

I received a call from my specialist and I could hear in her voice message she was sad for me. She said she was very sorry about the result, to return her call and to please take care of myself. I knew my specialist was trying all she could. When we spoke, she said she was disappointed and still believed she can achieve a pregnancy and it was just down to the right combination. She made a comment I've had a difficult run. I sure felt that way too. She was trying to squeeze in an appointment for me so I could start IVF on my next period, but she was all booked out. She had a phone consultation with me as she knew I just didn't want to wait around unnecessarily. We had a laugh together when I told her I was more stressed not doing IVF as it meant I was just waiting. She was a lovely lady, and she always gave me hope every time I visited or spoke to her to make a new plan for the next round.

Running parallel to the discussions with my specialist, I made an appointment with a brand new specialist to seek another opinion. This would become the third specialist I received information and advice from. It shocked him I'd eight implants with eleven embryos (plus two cancelled cycles to equal ten attempts). He requested my records from my specialist and advised if the tubes were absolutely blocked; he suggested removing them. I'd surrendered years ago that I wouldn't fall pregnant naturally. He told me I could have the tubes removed after an eight week wait to let my body recover from the last round. This meant I could only try IVF one more time this year and the funding assistance was due to be reduced by the Government the following January. I was grateful for this assistance as it allowed me to try more IVF attempts than I otherwise could have. There were still significant out-of-pocket expenses which I did not expect to be covered by anyone else other than myself as this was my choice.

I based all my decisions first on the medical requirements, but I also needed to factor any financial impact as I would somehow have to cover any gaps. I had another consultation with the specialist I had all bar the first attempt with. The specialist also ordered a blood test she hadn't requested before on this journey.

When I had the blood taken, I don't recall ever seeing so many vials of blood before in my life. I could feel the nurse changing bottle after bottle as the needle remained in my arm. I felt my head getting lighter and lighter and was certain I would pass out.

To this point, I believe we were working around the fallopian tubes. I now believed they needed to come out. My specialist called and offered a cancellation appointment. I was losing hope but still pushing through, somehow. I asked if she could take my tubes out and she advised that probably wouldn't make much difference but we could try, and that would have been her next suggestion. I said I was desperate and that I would try anything. I asked how long it would take for surgery. I told my specialist I'd seen another to get some clarity for my mind and whoever would book me in the quickest would be who I would go with.

I was in hospital three days later having my tubes removed with my original specialist. This would be my first of three sedations over the next five weeks. I was in pain when I woke from the laparoscopy surgery (through the belly button). I don't recommend this, but when I could move properly, I discharged myself from hospital at 8pm. I wanted something comfortable. I needed to get home. I wanted to sleep in my own bed.

I received some wonderful news from Ian and Rosalie, that my niece, Charlee was born and arrived safe and well on Friday 13th and that all my extended family were thrilled. While I wasn't able to have the connection of a pregnancy while Dad was alive, Rosalie and Ian were able to. Charlee was our connection to Dad. I was so happy. I was in the depth of isolation from my own world, but our whole family was so happy that a little girl joined us. I hoped she could somehow rub off on me and help me get my baby too. When I visited my new niece, Ian and Rosalie, through their moment of happiness, genuinely consoled me and said they will stand by me as I carry on giving it my all to become a mother. I thought this was the most beautiful and selfless act of compassion and felt I had tremendous family support. Although, I did not know if I would ever be standing where Rosalie was holding her precious baby.

I'm not sure I wanted to try again. I wanted a baby, but I'd now tried ten times. That is a high number of attempts through IVF. Maybe I just have to adjust to the fact I may never have my own child and enjoy the children in my family and my friend's children. I knew this was not what I wanted but I needed to process thoughts that were aligned with my reality. I wasn't getting pregnant. Then I got an email from Miss Sharp Shooter, Emma.

It read, "Good on you Jodes for trying again. Don't worry about how impressive the numbers are, you only need one embryo to work. Forget what happened last time as they have changed the treatment this time. It's a new start. Wait and see what the result of this cycle is.

If the clinic thought there was no hope, they will start discussing other methods. They haven't done this so hold on to hope my friend. People go through 8, 9, 10, 11, 12 rounds of IVF and they get a baby in the end (which is only a year so put it into perspective). They go through it so you can too, because you are stronger than anyone I know. You need to wipe the years it hasn't worked for you and start from today. Fresh start. You need to be positive, so get your bum into gear or I will have to come there and slap your bum for you! If you won't pull through, I will pull you through. This baby is coming whether you like it or not."

Good one Em! What are friends for!

Emma by this stage experienced two pregnancies and thanked me for being so supporting, knowing how difficult it was for me. Then Emma floored me. Emma offered to be a surrogate for me. What a selfless offer. I couldn't believe it. I have such beautiful friends. I thanked Emma immensely and said that I will try again. I said her third could be mine. My sister, who didn't have any children yet, also made me the same offer. What a sweetheart. I had it in me to try again. These kind and generous offers brought me hope and comfort that maybe one day I would have my own child, even if a different mumma carried for me.

I sat outside again for a while. I seemed to find peace there. The cockatoos and lorikeets would sit on the power lines at the back of my house. I hung a bird feeder up from the pear tree to attract the birds to enjoy some seeds. I had a hot chocolate on my wagon chair and concentrated on my breathing. I felt I could not go backwards, there was nothing to gain from letting the hurt penetrate through. If I didn't go forward, I would be left permanently stranded. I had eight negative results, two cancelled cycles and eleven embryos to date. I'd given all I had to get this far. All I had to do was try again, because after all, anyone that gets pregnant has to try.

I felt so far away from being a mum, but each attempt meant that wish could be just sitting around the corner ready to come true.

.

CHAPTER SIXTEEN

Forty Pregnancies

One of my most difficult experiences was the desire to have a child and not have one. I know this because this happened to me for ten unsuccessful IVF rounds. I was trying so hard to become a mother and everywhere I looked there were babies. There were babies in prams, babies in wraps, there were mothers just doting over their babies. One of my close friends fell pregnant while I was trying and didn't know how to tell me. She knew me well enough to just tell me but said it was extremely difficult for her to do.

I made myself a promise that I would be happy for anyone who got pregnant around me because I wouldn't wish what I was going through on anyone. I told my friend I wanted her to share all her happiness with me because my time will come one day. (Well, I'd hoped but was more convincing with my words to put my friend at ease to be open with me.) I explained I wanted her to share her experience with me as though

I wasn't going through IVF. I wanted her to have someone to lean on and I wanted our friendship to stay strong. I also was genuinely happy for my friend, after all it was her first child and she was thrilled. It did hurt. It did sting. But I chose to not feed the sad feeling and rise above it to find all the good thoughts.

A colleague invited me to her baby shower, and I was hurting so much. I didn't want to go, but I couldn't let myself do that. It would feel like I was giving in, but I also felt like I was entitled to as it was hard to be strong all the time. I always tried to choose the high road when faced with adversity, but this was really hurting me. I wanted to make a beautiful gift for the lady whose baby shower it was and I wanted to see her happy face when she opened the present and this is exactly what happened. This baby gave her life direction, and she was beaming with happiness.

It seemed the universe placed all the pregnant women in front of me to rub it in. I knew that wasn't the case, but they seemed to be everywhere. I felt like I was digging deep for strength and I hadn't recovered before I needed to search for strength again. Another friend needed to do IVF to conceive her first child. She asked me lots of questions and I explained the process. I'd three failed rounds by this point, so she was apprehensive about what lay ahead for her. I explained the injections in the stomach and she squirmed and I thought that is something you will have to quickly get used to. I was with my friend through her whole first round, through each ultrasound and most importantly, she called me to after she received the call from the nurse to advise me she was pregnant.

Yes, pregnant first attempt!

I was genuinely happy for her and wished her all the best and gave her a super strong hug. I didn't wish my three failed rounds on anyone because I was hanging out on a limb not knowing when this would end. Why would I wish that on anyone? She apologised to me for her outcome and I said I understand her kindness, but I asked her to be happy and keep supporting me and we can help each other. I wanted anyone I knew to get a positive result, and I hoped that one day that would be me. Having said all that, it really hurt. I wondered why I couldn't get a positive result, but knew I needed to keep going forward. No matter how I found the strength, I needed to keep going.

My wonderful brother Ian, and his equally superb fiancée Rosalie telephoned me, as we lived some distance away from each other. Ian and Rosalie knew my heartache. They, too, were supporting me through every single round of IVF.

They were sad for me when they wanted me to hear from them that they were pregnant again, so it didn't seem they were avoiding me or not supporting me. I could hear the sadness in both their voices. I explained they were bringing a beautiful child into the world who

AN IVF MIRACLE FROM MAHERS

would be my niece or nephew and I couldn't be happier. They accepted my congratulations but reiterated they were so proud of me for having the will to keep turning up despite the heartache. They said they would be there every step of the way and I have to say, I would be lost without them and their kindness.

My brother and I were close growing up and I could read my brother's sadness. I knew he wanted me to become a mother and would have given up anything he had in return for me to have a baby. Rosalie often cuddled me when I visited after an unsuccessful attempt. I could feel Rosalie wanted me to be a mother more than anything in the world. She was carrying her precious child and wanted me to as well but couldn't really push the issue as I'd been trying and it wasn't working. What I knew was this couple would never let me down.

Over the course of my pregnancy attempts, I counted forty pregnancies around me and each one stung. They were family members, best friends, friends and colleagues. Emma ended up having two children before me. All the pregnancies were right under my nose and it hurt me so much. I was crying on the inside but wanted to show these people I was happy because I was genuinely happy for them; I was just broken for me. Somehow, I found the courage to split my thinking into being genuine for their good news and dealing with my sadness. I refused to become bitter or not wish that people would get pregnant because that would

168

allow myself and my grounded morals to change and I wouldn't do that for anyone or anything. My parents taught me to be considerate of others and to respect myself and I could do both at the same time. These beautiful babies were nieces, nephews and friends' children and they gave me hope to stay strong and I adored them.

One friend said she understands if I didn't feel like visiting and I said I would as I didn't want to hibernate and let IVF totally change who I am. I don't know how I kept going.

I ended up not going to some baby showers. These were around the time when I felt emotionally weak. I didn't see the point in continually trying to prove anything to myself when I'd already done my best to go to the baby showers I could emotionally handle. I took each invite as it came and was kind to myself.

If I couldn't make it, I would send a present.

CHAPTER SEVENTEEN

What people say

Going through IVF is emotionally exhausting. People are an aspect of the IVF road to manage. People offer words of comfort, advice, and what they may feel is wisdom.

Having people around to support us in times of despair is wonderful and comforting. However, sometimes people's words don't have the impact they may have intended and are not helpful. Some people don't understand how mentally, emotionally and financially exhausting it all is. If only it was as easy as being positive.

Some people think what they're saying is the right thing, and it will make us feel better. Sometimes it may offer comfort, although at other moments, the timing of what they say does not reach us because we're feeling disconnected and isolated. Sometimes we completely dismiss what you've said as we look at you and wonder how you think what you're saying is helpful.

In the depths of despair, unfortunately, nothing anyone says can make it better. Only time can determine the outcome, and even then, you never forget.

I accept that genuine people's intentions come from an encouraging place for which is understood and appreciated and sometimes it may penetrate. Thank you for trying.

Following are some common statements I heard and others shared with me by IVF friends and those who have lost their little ones.

1. You need to relax.

2. Everything happens for a reason.

3. It's just not meant to be.

4. Just go on a holiday, don't think about it and it will work naturally.

5. It'll happen, just stay positive.

6. Hold my baby, it will make you feel better.

7. We have our rainbow (baby born following loss) and he has helped heal our hearts.

8. That you forget it all once you finally get a baby.

9. We are over-populated because of people like you who go through IVF to have a baby when clearly you weren't meant to.

10. If you have to go through all the hassle to have a baby, then it isn't meant to be.

11. What is your problem? It just worked for me.

12. I had my kids without even trying to fall pregnant.

13. Your struggle to be around other children is your issue. Get over it.

14. That it must be my fault (coming from non-medical opinionated people).

15. But you can try again soon.

16. Kids aren't the be-all and end-all.

17. Have you tried...? It worked for my son's teacher's soccer coach's wife.

18. That you're lucky you lost your baby sooner rather than later.

19. You are lucky to have the kids you have and that

losing a baby early in pregnancy wasn't meant to be.

20. In relation to first trimester miscarriages, is it really a baby anyway?

21. That good things happen to good people and bad things happen to bad people.

22. That maybe you just weren't supposed to be a mum.

23. That it's your fault because you 'chose' to start late.

24. That you're too old to be having any more babies.

25. That you're too fat or too skinny be a parent.

26. That you 'should be satisfied with one,' when you really yearned for four.

27. You're young. You've got plenty of time.

28. You chose to do IVF, so you have to put up with the pain.

29. If it's not meant to be naturally, why would you go through it?.

30. Keep trying, it will happen.

31. We didn't ask what you needed because we thought you'd have it all sorted.

32. After having a baby through IVF, so many people can naturally conceive their next child.

33. Don't worry, you'll definitely get pregnant, just keep trying naturally.

34. So, when are you having kids?

35. Why not adopt?

36. There are worse things that can happen.

37. Trust me, you're lucky you don't have kids.

38. Babysit my kids and you'll change your mind.

39. You put your career in front of having a family.

40. If you can't have children you'll have plenty of money. Work on Plan B.

It's difficult to relax with your life revolving around injections, hormones and being dictated by strict timelines. It is not proven that our perceived inability to relax can overcome nature and science.

I was dedicating all financial resources to creating a baby. There was no guarantee this financial investment would have a reward, yet it was a calculated risk to which I committed. There was no way I could go on a holiday because I had to be near the clinic for IVF appointments.

Following a negative pregnancy result and taking a forced break in order for my body to recover, I was trying to recover financially too. I said no to any holiday offers because I chose to try for a baby. A holiday was the last thing I could afford and needed to hear about.

Holding other people's children is a blessing and we are so grateful for these beautiful children in our lives, but no, it won't make me feel better. It tears my heart apart that I'm not holding my own baby (but I'm grateful you have yours).

It's not meant to be. This is just so hurtful. Who has the right to determine this for another person?

Anything that comes after 'at least' or 'you're lucky that' immediately made me switch off to what was being conveyed. There was nothing lucky about negative results and yes, I can see all the goodness around me for which I'm grateful. I still yearned for a baby.

If I'm talking to you about struggling to conceive, chances are we have tried almost everything at this point, but thank you for making suggestions when I'm so upset.

Everything happens for a reason was often said as a soothing or coping mechanism and in a sense to accept fate. Sometimes there can be nothing wrong and still no baby. So, the reason remains unknown and is not comforting.

Babies born after a loss don't negate the loss. One baby doesn't replace another. All losses hurt and everyone differs in how they cope with grief, even if a new baby comes along. You never stop grieving the missed opportunities and the (multiple) lost babies.

Yes, there are positives you can find in nearly every situation, but you still need the time and space to grieve and process the pain, even when you're in the middle of treatment.

I don't think some people understand the grief involved with infertility and treatment even before/ without pregnancy losses. You don't forget the torment. It changes you as a person, and your intervention and interpretation of this torment becomes your future. The new you.

Sure, more money would be available by not having a child through IVF, but it's not about money in the bank versus the desire to be a parent. If it was about saving money, I wouldn't have started.

And please, don't jokingly offer to donate your sperm or eggs, unless previously discussed. It's incredibly hard to accept our bodies sometimes can't do what we need them to, so confirming yours is useful and mine isn't and covering it as a joke, is not helpful.

Suggesting I should accept the outcome does not connect when I have invested so much emotionally, mentally and financially. I can only accept the outcome when money runs out, if I have medical evidence or facts that it won't work and then, I'm not sure I'm even ready to stop. Being a parent is the most important thing right now. So, don't take that away from me or try to talk me out of it, now or ever.

The desire to become a parent is likened to wanting to be the small percentage success story and beat the odds because that can and does happen. We know we are up against the odds, and it's a choice to start with these odds at each attempt.

How do you stop trying to become a parent when it is what your heart desires? When is enough, enough? Who determines this? Financial, medical, acceptance?

The following are some recommendations on how to approach and what you could say to an IVF patient to gently support them:

1. Be very sensitive.

2. Always think before you speak.

3. Your doctors sound like they know what they are doing.

4. I would love you to come to my baby shower, but will totally support your decision and there is no pressure from me.

5. Cook and deliver meals.

6. Ask what you can do to assist and truly listen for the answer.

7. Invite them somewhere and discreetly distract them from their own thinking.

8. Do not repeat their inner thoughts to others.

9. Let them know you care.

10. Research what they are going through.

11. Support males as well as females.

12. When suitable and if needed, encourage professional support.

13. Support their choices (to start, keep going, or stop IVF).

14. Offer to attend appointments as a support person.

15. Babysit their children so they can attend appointments.

16. Remember them on the painful days like Mother's and Father's Day.

17. Minimise the discomfort of your pregnancy within their presence.

18. IVF is not a taboo topic. Ask if your IVF patient wants to talk. They may need someone to vent to.

19. Admit your lack of IVF knowledge (if that's the case).

20. Research and understand some useful coping strategies and take a gentle lead.

Gentle support proved to be most effective with me as I was so incredibly upset on the inside and wore an invisible mask to carry on, on the outside.

CHAPTER EIGHTEEN

The King of Pop was gone

There'd been such a big build-up as usual to reach egg collection day. I was again sitting in pole position. I'd timed my trigger injection as requested thirty-six hours before my scheduled egg collection, to assist my eggs to release. I woke with so many nerves and butterflies in my stomach. It may seem I was becoming a professional at this routine, but deep down it took all I possessed to constantly coordinate this IVF world. Another needle, another surgery was all I could process.

Please, nothing go wrong on the way to the clinic, body of mine. Do everything you're supposed to. Please little eggs, please be ready.

I couldn't even contemplate not waking up from surgery and being told there were no suitable eggs.

Even thinking of this made me disconnect. My thoughts went numb, like I'd hit a wall and couldn't construct anything to get me through. I concentrated on breathing and tried to talk myself into being calm and do whatever I needed to do next. Just turn up Jodi. I'd sure proven I was effective at doing what needed to be done next. My job was to hold myself together in between these steps.

Today was different. Having a musical upbringing, today would hit me and I wasn't ready for it.

I grew up with Mum having music on all the time and Elvis was her all-time favourite entertainer. We've visited Graceland Memphis USA twice together. My Aunty Kathy rocks ACDC like no other woman I've seen and she sure proved this again when we watched ACDC in concert at Sydney in 2000. I would have to miss the next opportunity to see them in concert in February 2010 as I was thirty-eight weeks pregnant with Jy. It had been fifteen years since I'd been to the concert and I was mesmerised at the concert in Sydney, November 2015. ACDC opened the show with a video of man walking on the moon. Then a meteorite from the moon was plummeting to earth and when it landed, the stage lit up and the band appeared after the smoke cleared. What an absolutely brilliant concert! They sure do know how to rock. I still visit my brother now and he always has a new song to play for our family gatherings and they always have a great meaning.

My dad was a fan of country music and was once offered a recording contract after a record label executive watched him perform in a talent quest. It was a duet performance and the lady Dad sang with wasn't interested in the offer. I think this opportunity stayed in the back of Dad's mind forever, but it never stopped him singing or playing his guitar. He'd named me after a Gordon Parsons country music song called 'Jody'. Dad decided to spell my name with an I instead of a Y. I have wonderful memories of my dad singing this song to me. In September 2001, I wasn't in a financial position to fund the idea I had of surprising Dad. I borrowed the money from the bank as I figured I'd have time to pay it off as Dad may not be around long because of his age. I surprised Dad with an all-expenses paid holiday to Alice Springs and Uluru for Father's Day.

Our first event was a camel ride during a glorious sunset, which ended up at a delicious dinner. The following day we were walking past a pub named 'Bojangles' around 3pm and a band was playing. That's all Dad and I needed to hear. We went inside in and enjoyed the music. Dad went up to the singer on a break and asked if he could play a song. Next, I hear Dad over the microphone introducing the song for one special daughter, who brought him away on this holiday. Dad sang the song he named me after.

The crowd listened intently to the words and erupted at the end of the song. Everyone was then buying Dad beers so he was pretty happy (and tipsy). It was around

1am by this stage and I was yawning. I said, "Dad, do you think we should go back to our hotel?" thinking because of Dad's age at seventy-seven he might want to go to bed.

He replied, "I'm only just getting started, love!"

We both laughed.

Music ran through my family, and I was so sad the day I woke on 25 June 2009 to learn the super musician Michael Jackson was dead. I'd listened to him at school while constantly perfecting the moonwalk and watched him in concert in Sydney in 1996. The world was in shock. I was in shock. The music world was mourning. He was just too young and was about to start a comeback concert. It just wasn't fair. I wanted to sit and watch the news about this untimely story, but I needed to make my way to the clinic. There was so much riding on me arriving on time and surgery was booked for 10am.

I listened to the radio on the way to the clinic, trying to process the King of Pop was gone. I couldn't believe what I was hearing. I arrived at the clinic on time with my IVF bundle of nerves. The regular waiting room was cleared from the normal morning rush I was used to and it was just patients arriving for surgery at this time of the day. I changed into the surgery robe and sat bouncing my knee up and down in anticipation in the theatre waiting area.

Please, little eggs, please come out okay. Please one of them be the beginning of my baby. Please help me specialist, don't make any mistakes.

Here I was again. Taking a look around this old familiar place. The IVF theatre waiting room. There was food and a kettle and I was so hungry, but I was fasting and couldn't eat. I wondered if this would be the last time I would be here. I truly hoped so. I don't know how much more I had in the tank to keep doing this. Had I done everything that was expected of me, on time, every time? I believed I had. I believed there was no more I could have done to create a positive outcome. I'd given my all. This process I feared so much because of needles I was now quietly so grateful for. The nurse's voice distracted my wandering thoughts.

"Jodi, we're ready. Would you like to come in?"

I stood up hoping my nerves would allow my body to stay strong enough to hold me up because my legs felt weak. I did the familiar walk through the theatre doors and took a big breath. I said hello to my Fertility Specialist who was somewhat familiar with my pre-surgery nerves. The nurses were also used to me, but today our conversation turned to Michael Jackson. The medical staff even did a quick rendition of the moon walk, which made me laugh. We talked about what a talented man he was and how his music was part of history. The anaesthetist, who by the way, was a lovely reassuring man, had also experienced my pre-surgery nerves and said the right thing at the right time to settle me as best as he could. I couldn't look as the needle was inserted into the vein in my hand. I watched the vial of liquid ready to be connected to my hand and I knew soon I would be waking to hopefully the good news I did have some eggs. The anaesthetist said he was going to send me away on a holiday and to relax. That sounded pretty good to me at this point.

I remembered the big light above me turning into a swirling circle and I then realised I was waking up. Where was I? I was in a good sleep and I'm not ready to wake up now. Turn the lights off and let me sleep. As the medication wore off, I realised I was in the recovery bay and oh, that's right, I'm having eggs removed. Through a groggy state, I asked the nurse how many eggs they'd removed.

Please tell me there were some.

"Jodi, you have four eggs."

"How many?" I said.

"Four," she replied.

I dozed back off to sleep. Then I woke, not realising I'd already asked how many eggs I had and repeated myself. Finally, I was coming through the haze and remembered… I had four eggs. Wow! This means I have a chance. I've made it past the egg collection stage with eggs. I did it. Another stage cleared. I was proud of myself. I realised how strong I was, but this was testing me beyond my level of comprehension about what emotionally strong meant. The pain of having been here before and seeing a whole cycle through with a negative pregnancy test, not just once, but eight other times played in the back of my mind. But my theory was each time was a new chance. I had to grab on to the positive and believe that this really was a fresh opportunity. These thoughts had to be at the forefront of my mind. I needed to do whatever it took to block away the sadness of the journey so far so I was in the present moment completely. Maybe my baby is under construction. I hoped with everything I had that my baby was as I didn't want to come back and do this again. Ever.

I made my way home and relaxed for the rest of the day. I went into my baby's room and hoped that within a year, there would be sounds of joy filling the walls of the home. I was so ready for this child. I whispered in my baby's room, "I have done everything I can, please come to me now."

I went back to work the day following surgery to focus on the life I had outside yet running parallel to IVF while waiting nervously for the next step to jump through. I needed to return to normal knowing there was a potentially a life, potentially my child's life being created in a dish in the clinic twenty minutes from home. The normal wait any other person who conceives a child has to wait, that's what I had to do. It was just more transparent and regimented. Yet the difference for me was I would find out today if my eggs fertilised overnight into an embryo. Couples conceiving naturally don't get this level of information at this point. It's normally another eleven days before a couple conceiving unassisted gets the first indication via a pregnancy urine test. The sting of the result was weighing heavy on my mind for one of my previous rounds at this exact point in the cycle where the outcome was the egg did not fertilise. This meant that was the end of the cycle and it was as abrupt as that. The waiting to get to day one of a cycle, all the needles, ultrasounds and blood tests was for no gain, there was no chance of a baby this time around. How would I cope if the outcome was the same this time? More so, would I cope? I doubted myself.

The decision was made, I just didn't know the outcome, and the wait was torture. I resisted the urge to call the clinic prior to the agreed time. I tried to focus hard on my work to pass time.

It was time to call, and my fingers were shaking as I dialled the number. Please answer the phone. I spoke to a nurse who advised two of my four eggs fertilised. Thank goodness! The relief was overwhelming as some were still viable, but I'd gone from a 100% chance to 50% in two days. How can this be? Why didn't two eggs make it? I still don't know. But at this moment, the relief was overtaking the questions. I still have a ticket in this raffle. The nurse advised to call back on day three to check the progress of cell development. If the result was good on day three, I would then be booked into surgery for the embryo implant on day five. I then carried on with my usual routine of going to work and protecting my body by resting for the next few days. I'd put my life on hold to this point and I believed protecting my body and resting was paramount to the success.

I found it difficult being caught in these days of waiting. In fact, the whole IVF experience is waiting. My embryos were in a clinic and I needed to wait two more whole days to get the next update. This was an unbearable wait.

I again watched the clock to ensure I did not call prior to the agreed time, even though the clinic may have known some time sooner. I needed to wait and wait I did. I again dialled the number preprogramed in my mind and spoke to a nurse. I got good at picking the tone of their voices to anticipate the news they may deliver me.

"Hi, it's Jodi Maher here, and I'd like to check the progress of my embryos please."

They advised my embryos were still viable and growing and that they were developing at the required cell rate. We were aiming for 100 cells by day five and were on track. My eyes welled with tears. I had made it to day three! This means I have crossed another huge milestone. The advice of the nurse was to take care of myself and please come in at an agreed time that we made for day five for implantation. I was given all my pre-surgery instructions (which I knew already from experience). I was stoked.

I hung up the phone at work and walked away from my desk and cried tears of relief and hope. I couldn't stop crying this time. I'd made it to day three, like eight other times before. It was hard to sit in a comfortable, happy place for too long before the uncertainty set in again. Why hadn't it worked in the ten rounds up until now? We slightly changed the formula each time. Had we changed it too much this time? How will I fill in the next two days? Go to work and carry on like everyone else, I guess. I just want the answer now! I knew full well I was in a vulnerable medical jail and I could get a phone call tomorrow on day four and be told the embryos didn't make the night, but so far so good. I was being booked into surgery for implantation in two days' time. Off I went to my boss to ask for another day off. He was very supportive and I had a lot of sick leave accrued, so he didn't have an issue with it being utilised for medical purposes.

Every time my phone rang, I didn't want it to be the clinic as that might be heartrending bad news. Mum called me at this point and I answered and said, "Phew, thank goodness it's you Mum."

What if human error at the clinic now meant I would lose my embryo I fought so hard for? Because people make mistakes, right? I went for a walk at lunch to clear my mind, but the worry of things outside my control kicked in. What if the electricity failed at the clinic? I then remembered they had backup generators. This thought somehow soothed me. I knew I wouldn't rest easy until they'd implanted the embryo and it was 'on board'.

I didn't expect work to make allowances for me, but I was so tired. I arrived at work on day four drained, but I did my best at work as I owed it to my employer who'd given me so many days off work for IVF. I just hoped this good will and support would continue and it did.

As day four came to a close, I went to bed that night and was restless. My mind couldn't help but wander. What happened if the scientist made a mistake and matched the wrong sperm and egg and it's now too late? Did they label the egg and sperm correctly? That couldn't possibly happen to me, could it? I'd read a book about this happening and I bet that couple thought it would never happen. They would have just been like me, trusting that humans and machines were doing their job. Had my embryos survived today? Were they still growing right this minute? Will I wake to a call to say don't come in for your implant as your embryos sadly didn't make it? I tried to switch off all the what if thoughts and focused on the facts. As far as I knew, and last heard as of yesterday, was that I had two strong embryos which I desperately needed to make it through the night.

Hold on little embryos at the clinic, your mummy is coming to get you.

Maybe tomorrow is the day I get pregnant.

CHAPTER NINETEEN

Two Embryos and an eleven-day Wait

I woke feeling weary. I was so tired from a broken night of sleep, but I was excited. This was one of the most exciting days to reach in the cycle. The other I imagined was hearing a nurse tell you that you were pregnant. (So unromantic!) I again fasted and made my way to the clinic for my scheduled implant. I did the familiar drill of chatting to the reception staff, changing for surgery and bouncing my leg in anticipation of what was to come. I was wondering what food I would eat when I woke up again. I'd convinced myself through all the surgeries how to cope with needles. Rather than worry about them, (which didn't stop the dreaded anticipation of getting one), I would be grateful to get some extra sleep when I was knocked out as I was so tired. I believed my body and mind was just pushing through day after day through the tired haze IVF had become for me. It just all seemed to roll from one needle to another with not much time in between.

This time though I was about to have a conversation that could have changed the outcome that is my world today.

I understand the law has changed now for singular embryo implants, but back when I undertook IVF, there was room to move and it was a case-by-case decision made by my specialist. I was informed of the grade of the embryos which included how many cells my two embryos had and advised me she would implant the better of the two. This immediately didn't sit well with me and not being one to go against my gut feeling, I respected my specialist's position but questioned this decision. I accepted the explanation of the second embryo being a lower grade, but if I was to ever speak about it; it had to be right now.

To show respect, I said I heard the reasoning, but to this point, I'd had endless needles in my stomach, about one hundred and fifty blood tests, and numerous ultrasounds. The idea of implanting one embryo and halving my chance by freezing the other for use at a later date was something I could just not process or comes to terms with in that moment. I knew I'd no idea where to find the money for the next round, should there be one. (I hadn't finished this round and was gearing up for the next one.) So, I was throwing everything at the round I'd paid money for a pregnancy from today's round.

I was about to face my eighteenth operation/ sedation (third in five weeks). I'd paid money towards this long and tedious process, had days off work, forgone gatherings with family and friends and put my life on hold. Not giving what I thought was every chance I could seemed like I was doing half a job and I'd not done that at any point of this IVF journey and I wouldn't start now. No way, not after all these years, not after the sheer determination and resilience I'd displayed. No way!

I explained that I desperately want a child and regardless of a single child or multiple birth, boy or girl, disabled or abled, I would accept whatever I am given. I said I was tired and needed a break from coming here and doing this time and time again. That I needed something to give to commence the next stage of my life which was to be a mum. I asked to be given every chance I have available today, right here, right now. I was not rude, but I was firm and showed the utmost respect for her position, and then stepped down off my emotional soap box.

I watched for a reaction on the specialist's face, hoping my academy award speech connected. I could see she was considering my plea via her facial expressions and said she will be back in a moment.

Please specialist, hear my plea. Give me every chance I have now.

I became anxious. The specialist returned and said she will implant two. It worked! She'd heard my plea and granted my wish. We were implanting two embryos. I then relaxed knowing I was giving this 100%. I'm a big believer of asking. You don't know unless you ask. No was an option as the answer, but yes could also have been and in this case it was. This answer was about to change my life.

I was so hungry but knew the food I would have on the other side of my next anaesthetic would be delicious even if it was toast in recovery. A nurse I knew well called me into theatre and said I was nervous. She said I've done this before and she knows I'll be right and it won't take long and I'll be in recovery. I again said hello to all the familiar staff in the theatre and my lovely anaesthetist took care of me and my nerves straight away.

My specialist showed me a picture of my two embryos up on the monitor. I had a moment to myself where I wished upon a falling star that it would bless me with a child or children this time around. I really was on a limb and if my options were to fall or fly, I wanted to fly. I was so sad from the setbacks. I said to the little embryos that I am ready and please stay with me this time. There were butterflies in my stomach and I laid down on the bed and saw the big light above me swirl as they sedated me.

I woke up in recovery and this time I wasn't sure through my groggy state if I'd had eggs removed or embryos implanted. Under sedation and coming out of it confused me and I remember asking the nurse how many eggs I had removed and then fell back asleep. I asked the same question when I woke again and remembered as the nurse advised they implanted two embryos today and everything went well. I took a big deep breath and sighed with relief. It was a real milestone to reach having an embryo implanted. I'd made it! From this point, I couldn't do anything more that was expected of me. The embryos would either work or they wouldn't and from this moment on I had no control.

I made my way home and rested for the remainder of the day and commenced the anxious eleven-day wait for the pregnancy result day.

The following day I went back to work and tried to give it my full attention. I'd been so impressed with the support of my employer, but without their support it would have been much more difficult to juggle my medical and work world. If only they knew how hard it had been. While I was at work, I tried to give 110% effort to repay the kindness and support I'd received.

I became close to a lady named Kim at work who was also going through IVF and a few weeks earlier had the difficult task of advising me she'd become pregnant. Kim was worried how to inform me. Kim advised me she had some news she wanted to share and would rather it come from her and advised me she was pregnant. I was delighted for Kim and had a speech ready in my mind for people who felt awkward advising me of their pregnancy, knowing the difficulty I was having. I truly was happy for Kim as I sure do know how hard it was to fall pregnant through IVF, so any person who could, I was happy for them. I also knew Kim experienced several miscarriages, so this

197

was wonderful news. It gave me hope it may work for me one day and I hoped with all I had this little baby would hold on for Kim.

There was always a sting of sadness when someone else told me they were pregnant, but my mindset was to be delighted for them and show them that. I kept the sadness of *will it ever happen* to me inside and processed it myself. It sure did hurt like crazy to learn of other pregnancies. It wasn't my time, it was theirs, and I needed to dig deep to believe that and carry on.

Two days after they implanted the embryos, I looked at the list of jobs I wanted to finish around the house prior to a baby arriving and staining the timber deck was one of them. I got everything ready and then called the clinic to check if this was something I should be doing. They encouraged me to not do any staining just in case I was pregnant. I'd a feeling to check, but I also wanted to keep my life outside IVF running along too.

I found the eleven-day wait to be a nervous yet welcome distraction as I knew I'd a chance as the embryos had implanted. It was nice to catch my breath again and not have to go to the clinic for any needles, blood test results or ultrasounds. It was almost like enjoying the calm before a storm, or it could have been the beginning of another let down.

I almost felt like I had to jump outside of my body for a while, but this just wasn't possible. The constant, every day commitment was wearing me down and I was so tired. I needed a break. I was having the required breaks in between treatment cycles, but the mental commitment didn't stop when the physical breaks did. This was years' worth of tiredness I was feeling today. I was carrying a heavy load and it exhausted me. I went to bed early that night and fell into the deepest sleep out of fatigue.

When I woke, I felt refreshed, and I reflected on what I'd done to get to this point and I truly amazed myself. No wonder I hit a wall with tiredness the night before. I longed for this process to be over but I knew if I didn't do the next step, there would be no baby. No matter what that meant or what tiredness I felt or obstacles before me, I had to push through. I needed to find a way and do it. I tried hard to keep positive and think of strategies to deal with the anxiety of the wait and wonder. I focused on my nutrition and water intake and thought about the joys of being a mum. This scared me to think this, because if it didn't work I'd allowed myself to think in a place I so desperately wanted to be in, I would have to then come back from there. I'm a big believer in not denying myself and by not thinking of that happy place would be just doing that. I would rather pick myself up from a fall than be stagnant and hide real feelings.

After a sleep to rejuvenate and two-day weekend ahead of me, I drove three hours to visit one of my biggest fans, my mum. When I arrived, Mum gave me the biggest cuddle and spoilt me for the next two days by just looking after me. Just what the doctor ordered. I talked to Mum about her pregnancy journey and found a whole new appreciation for my mum. My mum told me about how her mum (my nan) had seven children. We discussed how lucky I was to have the luxury of IVF and if I were from a previous generation, I wouldn't have the chance to try to have a child/ren. I often stopped to silently thank IVF. The creation of this gift to bless people with a baby was something I was just constantly amazed by.

I felt like I was letting my support network down. I know deep down this wasn't the case but part of me felt sad when I looked at my people and could see they were trying to be strong for me when they were hurting too. I knew they wanted a grandchild, a niece or a nephew, or a cousin, but we all knew how life goes and this was out of my control.

My Aunty Kathy phoned me and said she was very proud of how I was handling this situation. She couldn't fathom how difficult this was for me and what I was going through emotionally but would continue to keep me strong. She always treated me like a daughter and encouraged me to take care of myself and said she knew the fighter in me would keep trying.

Cathy at work was aware I was in the midst of the eleven-day wait and had been with me during this process long enough to know I wasn't done yet even if this result was another negative. She observed me rolling up my sleeves, so to speak, getting ready for round twelve. Cathy told me this many years later. I don't remember doing this, but knowing my inner strength to get a baby, it certainly sounded like me.

CHAPTER TWENTY
The Phone Call

The day of finding out a pregnancy result for a couple who can conceive without IVF, I imagine, would be so exciting. You buy the pregnancy test and conduct the test at home. After a few minutes all will be revealed, hopefully seeing two lines appear on the test stick. This is how I imagined it would be for me. Not that the IVF pregnancy result day wasn't exciting, it just felt so clinical. Well, after the number of rounds I'd completed, it sure felt this way. I was used to how clinical IVF felt a long time ago, yet it always sat so strangely and just not the way I wanted to conceive a baby.

On 11 July 2009, eleven days after they implanted the two embryos, I woke much earlier than the sleep in I'd planned. It was the anxious side of me wanting to face the day as this is the day I'd committed to eight weeks of the last IVF cycle for the pregnancy result day. I sighed in relief I'd made it to today and it wasn't a dream as I'd dreamt before only to wake and be disappointed.

I didn't feel well. I was exhausted and felt like my period were definitely coming and I hadn't got out of bed yet. Trying to interpret my body and whether my period would beat the pregnancy phone call from the nurse at noon on result day was a race to see which would win. After checking my period hadn't arrived, I smiled at the prospect of still being in the race. I took a breath and thought, please don't come, not today, not before I have a baby. This was the only indicator I could go by. During the whole IVF cycle, I'd not used a do-it-yourself pregnancy test kit at home. I just couldn't face it. I didn't want to have to see a negative result (which had been my IVF journey so far) and hope it was wrong. I'd shut down to this method of finding out the result. The wait felt agonising today. I didn't even know how to feel anymore. I am at a crossroads of hope and despair. I know it can go either way today.

Feeling pregnant and feeling like you are getting your period brings the same cramps and the uncomfortable feeling of being bloated. I just couldn't tell what my body was doing, although I was certain I wasn't pregnant based on my cramping stomach and sore breasts.

I wasn't hungry at all but decided on the chance I was carrying my little one (or two), I would continue to do the basics for me. Which was to eat well and drink lots of water. IVF trained me to drink 2.4 litres a day, something I couldn't drink a lot of before, so I ate to keep my metabolism going.

It was pregnancy result day, but I was feeling cranky, tired, lost and annoyed. Why had I made it so far and was feeling so detached and defeated for? I felt alone and trapped in this body that wouldn't produce a baby and here I was hanging on to what felt like the slimmest odds again, like so many times over the years. Not one to be negative and I can find the good in almost anything, but I just felt the process was still spinning around like a broken record for me.

I felt annoyed and convinced I would soon get my period. I didn't feel well and was upset when I thought of the crushing feeling I'd experienced so many times before when I reached this day. In fact, this was the ninth pregnancy result day during my eleven cycles. (One cycle was cancelled before the eggs were collected because of overstimulation and the other was cancelled the day following egg pick up when none of my eggs fertilised overnight.)

I had to fill in my time so I did some housework and couldn't stop thinking and overthinking. In fact, never has the saying 'never judge a book by the cover' rung so true. I looked fine on the outside, but I was a mess on the inside. I battled between staying positive, which I had done on this day so many times before, right up until the shattering phone call from the nurse.

This time though, I'd given up. I can normally use the power of a strong mind to keep going but I think the reality side kicked in. I surrendered to the possibility that while today could be a good result, as I'd abruptly felt so many times before, it could also bring a result I did not want.

Looking back now, I think it was my way of starting the letdown phase before the outcome was known so I could somehow help myself fall down more slowly and gently rather than a sudden thud. It was a different technique and thought process to all my other result days, but obviously was what I could muster at the time. You see, I like to stay strong and positive, but I realised I am only human and the strength and resilience I'd displayed to date, took a tremendous amount of will and determination. I don't feel the words, 'broken heart' does justice to the devastation of a negative result on an IVF pregnancy result day. I also feel that it's unrealistic to hide real feelings for too long. I was sad and I was defeated, so I just let myself be in this place for a little while knowing it would pass. Giving up is something that doesn't come easy for me and this moment was hard for me because I felt I'd let myself down in a way but I needed to let go.

I believe people have hardships in all walks of life and today, this was one of mine and I was facing it head on. I was certain I was not pregnant. I thought I've waited around before on this day and could have been getting jobs done around the house. I was feeling sad, anxious, confused but also empowered because I released the feelings of expectations and the feeling I wanted to feel the most was to be happy and pregnant. I felt trapped and wanted to somehow escape the emotions I was feeling and just sleep or do something, anything.

It was 10.30am, and I went to the garage and started unpacking some boxes. Given my rare negative mindset I was in, I started moving boxes around and convinced myself it was okay, but soon after I couldn't ignore the gut feeling. I decided I should just wait a few more hours and common sense prevailed. I left cleaning out the garage on the list of jobs I just couldn't do while in creating a baby phase. Nothing was worth the risk of doing anything silly now.

I was really struggling today. I worried I may fall into an uncontrollable sob if it didn't work today the way I so desperately needed it to. I didn't know how much more I could take. How would I cope? More so, would I cope? I didn't want to hear it again that I wasn't pregnant. That news had beaten me up so many times. I got back up again and I wanted to stay up and keep going up. It crossed my mind of how I would pay for the next round if the news wasn't good today. I changed my thinking to just be in the present moment, just deal with one step at a time. I thought of Mum and the guidance she would have given me and that settled me down. Even though I felt like I'd walked thousands of steps and each one of those one at a time, I felt my mum's wisdom and it comforted me. So, I parked the worry of the finances for the next round and walked out to the backyard. The one thing I knew about my powerful ability to think positively was that even though I was juggling emotions and I was feeling down, I wouldn't be unpacking and staying there long.

The sun was shining; it was a glorious day. The birds were flying in the back yard and a cockatoo and rainbow lorikeet landed on the power lines as they often did. I felt warm and cosy and became lost in the thought of being a mother. I allowed myself to fantasise about what my child would look like. What features of mine would he or she have? I pictured my little one learning to walk in the backyard and tumbling over and getting back up again and a smile came to my face. Focusing on these beautiful thoughts settled me down from the agitated and upset phase I was in. I was packing up those bags and moving out of negative town.

I concentrated on my breathing, which is something I did when I felt I'd no control. At least I could control my breathing. What if my little one was really on board? I wondered about all the joy this child would bring to my life.

I went for a walk into the room that would become my baby's room and felt so happy at the thought of this room being filled by the sounds of a beautiful baby. It also scared me so much that maybe I would never become a mother and it felt like such a waste of a mother's heart who would become one of the most devoted mothers.

I went back outside to do some light gardening and then decided I would just sit and do nothing and the serenity of that would help me leading up to the phone call.

I sat on my favourite wagon chair that Dad and I used to sit on and I wondered how he would feel now if he were still alive. What would he be saying to me? I knew it would be simple and would connect with me and it would have been something like, "Hang in there, I know you can do this."

I was taking in everything nature was offering around me. The pear tree was bare from the winter season and there was a chill in the air. There were leaves of beautiful colours on the ground. I looked to the cloud formation in the sky and tried to see if I could make out the shape of a baby. I noticed the cracks in the wagon chair and that it was overdue to be stained. I was feeling more relaxed in the mind, but my body felt like it was shaking on the inside and I felt a little weak.

It was now 11.30am and the butterflies in my stomach were constant. I felt like I would be sick from my nerves, so I kept concentrating on my breathing techniques. I could have already been pregnant and didn't know it. I smiled at the thought of being given the news I'd desired for so long. Would this phone call be the call that changes everything? I sure hope so. Again, I felt I'd done everything that was expected of me medically. I felt proud and comforted knowing there was nothing more I could have done.

Was everything I surrendered on this journey so far going to be worth it today? You see, I believe you reap what you sow. I said no to many things along this journey. Some were catching up with friends who lived interstate as I needed to remain home and near the clinic for medical tests over the weekend. The other was because all my money had gone to IVF and I couldn't afford other things. All choices I made willingly to have a baby. I believe we can't have everything we want all the time, but I do believe in backing up and trying your best. I really wanted this baby and the sacrifices I'd made so far and the desperation of needing to hear good news was making me teary.

I called Mum to share my current feelings and Mum said it wasn't long now and I'd done an amazing job to get this far and she was proud of me regardless of the outcome. I said I was feeling so nervous and Mum said she loved me very much. Mum later told me she didn't know what to say to me but offered me the support she could.

I started pacing around the backyard and was

watching the time count down. It was now 11.50am and in ten minutes' time, I would know. I was looking at the flowers and tried to make ten minutes feel like one, but it felt like one hundred. I was quiet in my solidarity. I felt as calm as I could be, but my heart was racing. I no longer had any control over that. I felt a shift in me, that somehow if this doesn't go my way today, the fight is over. I can't take anymore. I'm trying to soften my grief by appreciating what I do have in my life. Gratitude was my way to heal. The grief resurfaced. The hope was taking over. I still hadn't got my period. My hopes were rising. I hoped my pregnancy levels were too.

The nurse would now know if I was pregnant as she would have to gather her records to call me. It was 11.55am, and I was sitting down staring at my phone. Just waiting and waiting. Something I felt I'd done for so many years now. It was now two years, two months and twenty-eight days since I first started IVF and had completed eleven back-to-back rounds in that time. It was now down to this moment. The time was 11.58am, and I was holding my phone with both hands, waiting and hoping the nurse wouldn't be delayed.

I felt my phone vibrate and looked at the screen to recognise a number that I'd memorised so well. The

IVF clinic was calling me now! My heart felt like it skipped a beat and my mouth went dry and I took a big deep breath. I answered the phone in a quivering nervous tone and said hello.

The nurse said, "Hello Jodi, its Shiralee."

And I knew in that moment I was pregnant. I'd become in tune with the nurses and in particular Shiralee's tone as she'd called me four out of my nine pregnancy result days, plus many other times to advise me the outcome of tests. My intuition told me I was pregnant by the four words that she'd just spoken. I hoped I was picking up the right vibes and hope is such a powerful feeling, but I just didn't want it to come crashing down on me now. Then Shiralee uttered the words I'd laid everything on the line for.

"I have some great news, Jodi. You are pregnant!"

My eyes welled with tears and I put my hand to my mouth in shock and said, "Oh that is just the most wonderful news, thank you so much, I'm so happy. Are you sure?"

Shiralee laughed and responded in a delighted voice. "Yes, I'm sure, Jodi. You are pregnant."

Well, I lost it! I couldn't stop crying. This was the moment I'd been waiting for. It had finally arrived. I immediately pictured myself as the most devoted mother and knew I would do whatever I could to make this work from here on in. I asked what the Human Chorionic Gonadotropin level was and she said it was in the hundreds. As I knew a positive pregnancy test was higher than fifty, this was immediate confirmation my hormone level meant I was p-r-e-g-n-a-n-t! I felt like a blubbering mess. Shiralee congratulated me again, then encouraged me to rest and advised me to call my obstetrician on Monday and make an appointment in three weeks' time for a seven-week check-up.

I hung up the phone and did a little dance. I was absolutely thrilled. I was pregnant, my baby was on board and it was my job now to ensure I protected this little one every step of the way. I thanked my little one for staying with me and said we can do this together and to stay strong. The body I once felt had let me down had now shown me it could create my baby. I immediately began my mother instincts and would go on to protect my baby like a mother tiger would her cub, just like my mum had with me. I walked away with a little pregnant waddle and my hand on my stomach.

People generally wait until the twelve-week

pregnancy timeframe to advise friends and family. However, my personal choice was to let my support network know straight away. They'd all been on this roller coaster with me which seemed to have more downs than ups and I wanted to finally give them the good news they have hoped for, for me. I didn't want to deny them or myself the chance to enjoy the coming weeks of being pregnant as I wouldn't get the time back and if all went well until the twelve-week mark. I anticipated I'd feel we've all missed many opportunities to be delighted together. It was a risk, but I'd proven I was a risk taker and started making my calls.

I called Mum, and she answered.

"Hello Jode, how did you go, love?"

I responded with tears and realised that was how I'd been with Mum when I called before with negative pregnancy results. I just cried and couldn't get my words out.

Mum said, "Oh Jode."

I could tell she thought I wasn't pregnant and after the silence of trying to construct words I said, "Mum, I'm pregnant!"

There is something about a mother that cries. As a child you feel your mother's sadness and it often upset me whenever I'd seen my mum cry before. This time she cried and cried and she too was trying to speak but couldn't!

Mum finally said through her tears, "Jode, that's wonderful news. I'm so happy for you, well done, I'm so proud of you my baby girl, you did it!"

I was so happy. We shared our delight together, and I eventually got myself together again. I knew I would cry telling Mum either result as the release of emotion had a direction to travel, which was either sad or happy and both made me cry, either shattering or pure delight. Mum said I was made of the right stuff referring to my strength to constantly back up all the time. She said she was so proud of my determination and said she will be here to support me the whole way.

I called other family and friends, notably Ian, Rosalie, Renée, Emma, Peita and Aunty Kathy to share the exciting news and as you can imagine, everyone was thrilled. I couldn't wait to call every one of them. One reaction was one I would have to censor if written in this book!. I was listening for the delight in their voices and I heard it. I finally felt that I could put my support crew out of their misery. I could finally let them know I was pregnant. This was my time to shine. I'd gone beyond the call to get to this point in time and was so proud of what I'd achieved.

I walked back into my baby's room with a huge smile on my face. I looked around at how I may decorate the room and thought about sewing and craft projects for my little one.

I was on a high for the rest of the day. So many other times sadness filled the second half of the day, but not today. I'd finally got that phone call I'd desired for so long. I kept replaying the phone call in my mind and got emotional. I was pregnant and what a battle it had been to get this far.

It had been a big day and there was a precious baby on board (f-i-n-a-l-l-y) and as the day ended; it was now time for me to have what I hoped would be the best sleep I would have in a long time. Every move I will make from this day onwards would be to protect my baby and myself. It was now time to sleep, only this time, there were two of us.

Good night, my little one (or two).

CHAPTER TWENTY-ONE

My growing tummy and glowing face

I don't know why IVF worked on the eleventh round. I can only speculate that maybe the tubes were releasing a fluid that was poisoning the environment and the embryos couldn't develop. That, or it was a different medical recipe, or both. I still don't know and probably never will.

I often had these fleeting moments where I questioned whether the pregnancy was real. It was so surreal. It was strange to be in my body that couldn't somehow be pregnant to being in the same body that could. And it took me many months to settle into feeling safe with this pregnancy. I was petrified it would be taken away from me. At the same time, I couldn't believe the heavy burden of trying to get a positive pregnancy result had lifted. Had I really received that phone call advising I was pregnant or was it a dream?

I moved from the waiting world of IVF to a different wait, and this pregnancy wait was as nerve-wracking at times. Although now I was just like any other person who conceived naturally or with assistance and needed to hope that all would progress well.

I really didn't like needles and never got used to them after all these years; the fear of each needle still startled me. Given I had so many through IVF, I was thrilled to stop the stomach injections. That would be one less thing to remember to do every day. They advised me soon after that as a precautionary measure I needed to inject a needle every day of my pregnancy in my stomach to prevent blood clotting. I was taken back because I'd already celebrated not having to have any more needles in my stomach.

At times like this, I often grounded myself by thinking there were people who had medical conditions that required them to do things others squirm at. People with diabetes adapt to injecting many needles as their life depends on it. I thought of people who couldn't stop and had permanent medical plans. While it didn't minimise my fright of this news, I quickly put it into perspective and was grateful for the medical care

I was receiving to protect this precious child of mine. I gathered some momentum from my imaginary tank of strength, topped it up, took it in my stride and did what had to be done. Another day, another needle!

My friends often called to check in with me. They told me they were still in shock. I must admit, I was too. I was pregnant. I felt the stress of being committed to IVF leaving me, and it was such a release. I was a bunch of different emotions. I just needed my baby to stay with me. Emma said I have had a huge emotional and physical lead up to this point so she can understand why I am so tired and worried.

I could not stop smiling when I checked the letter box and received a congratulations letter from my clinic confirming my pregnancy. This reached me in a beautiful way. I was reading in writing that I was pregnant and it confirmed in my mind on a whole new level. They included information regarding local support networks during and beyond pregnancy. This was helpful as I'd no idea of what community networks were available.

At seven weeks I was talking to my friend Emma about how lethargic and sick I was feeling. Emma made me feel better.

"Constantly feeling sick and tired gets you down. Add to that, huge amounts of different hormones and all the stress of IVF, not getting pregnant and losing your dad. It is no wonder you are drained. And that is okay. You are entitled to feel that way… but it will get better. Another few weeks and it will start to subside. Are you able to eat any more yet? I am looking forward to your call or text tomorrow and hope and pray everything is well. I think it will be. You will be amazed at seeing your bub and it will give you a nice lift."

I lost my appetite and wasn't sure if this was normal, but I made sure I continued to eat at least three meals and three healthy snacks a day to keep my metabolism balanced.

Amanda was at work in another part of the building and called me. I could sense in her voice there was something important she needed to tell me. She said she didn't know how to and I asked her to just say what it was. I knew already what it was as I'd heard this approach many times before. But this time instead of rolling with my pre-rehearsed speech of compassion, understanding, support and my time will come, I had the same news to share. Amanda advised me she was pregnant and was treading lightly with the conversation and I could tell was leading up to sharing her compassion it hadn't worked for me when it had for her.

Normally I wouldn't interrupt such wonderful news, but I needed to stop Amanda. Amanda could not believe what she was hearing. Neither could I. We'd both conquered a positive pregnancy result and what a battle it was for both of us. We met up in the building and had a congratulation cuddle. When I originally met her, I thought she'd something going on as she seemed like she was under pressure and it didn't seem to leave her. I later found out she was riddled with IVF medication and was desperately trying to expand her family and then I understood. We both bonded over supporting each other. Amanda was an inspiration for me at work and I have fond memories of shedding wonderful tears on this day.

I explained to Emma now I'm off the hook with IVF I feel I will get my life back a little (not that the commitment wasn't worth it). I was grateful for the feeling of freedom from the medical process year after year. I thanked Emma for her support and explained it had been such a big build-up and I don't know how I did it. I was determined, but it was taking its toll on me. I was so exhausted. Let's hope we make it through the ultrasound tomorrow.

The next day was my first pregnancy appointment with my specialist at seven weeks. It was such an exciting moment. Every appointment from this day on would be constant amazement. Each appointment meant I was getting closer to meeting my child. Walking into the waiting room, I did not know what to expect as I would find out if there was a heartbeat and if so, how many. I was so concerned and worried I would be told there wasn't a heartbeat. I wasn't focusing on the worst-case scenario, but it is a worry of any pregnant woman facing the first ultrasound. I accepted there was nothing I could do other than accept whatever news they gave me. I was excited and secretly hoped I would be having twins and given two embryos were implanted, this was a strong possibility with my family history of twins. The specialist commenced the ultrasound, and I waited with an elevated heart rate, hoping she would say good news and my wish was granted. My specialist had a comforting manner and worked as quickly as possible as she would have known I was sweating on the outcome. There was one heartbeat and all the measurements were as expected. I could hear the comfort in my specialist's voice and this made me relax in a way I never really could, until now. This little baby was still with me and I was ecstatic. My specialist advised me to make an appointment with an obstetrician to monitor my pregnancy. There were so many defining moments of my baby becoming a reality and this was one of them. The walk out of that surgery was such a huge relief. I'm sure I was floating with delight.

The Swine Flu epidemic broke out in Australia in these early weeks of my pregnancy and it concerned me. The doctors considered pregnant women high-risk cases for catching this flu. I'd woken at 5am feeling sick and wondered if I had Swine Flu. It turns out I didn't, but I was on high alert to protect my pregnancy and doing everything right was my mission at this point in time. Nothing else came close. I worked so hard to get to this point. As all women wish for, I was just hoping that everything would be okay and I would reach the twelve-week mark. I booked in for this ultrasound and the images mesmerised me on the screen. They explained each image and I just couldn't believe it. They told me everything looked fine, and I took the biggest deep breath. This was a milestone I was secretly wishing for ever since I found out I was pregnant. I felt like I was gaining solid momentum that I would make it to the end with a healthy pregnancy.

I felt so sick with nausea from six to sixteen weeks and all I could focus on was work, eating well and drinking water. One morning I started work at 7am and knew I needed to make it until 3pm before I could leave. I'd no idea how I would do it and the thought of backing up again tomorrow was exhausting, but I did it. I walked in the door at 3.20pm and went to bed until the next morning for a 7am start. The tiredness was severe, and the nausea was terrible. The only way I found relief was to graze on food and the nausea left me for just a little while (before it abruptly returned). It took until week sixteen for it to finally sink in that I really was pregnant and I didn't need to go back to IVF. Around this time my sickness was only present in the evenings. It was such an empowering feeling and every day I felt the gift of being pregnant. The miracle of life is such a gift. What a blessing it is.

When I was fifteen weeks pregnant, I set up the nursery with Mum. It was such a magical time. I was taking it all in and had butterflies in my stomach from excitement. I purchased my friend Peita's nursery furniture. It didn't seem necessary or resourceful to buy anything else as Peita took such good care of the furniture. It was a medium-stained timber and had a single bed, cot, toy box and shelf. I displayed a figurine on the shelf given to me by a special lady named Cathy who sat beside me at work during many negative results of IVF and my whole pregnancy. The figurine was a ceramic woman holding her pregnant stomach, and I absolutely adored this gift.

An ironic thing happened when Jy was four years old. A circle of friends gave each other a random gift. I chose a lovely lady named Tanya and made her and her family a set of embroidered towels and she gave me the matching ceramic figurine to the pregnant lady. Only this time it was a young boy. I'd wanted this figurine for some time but hadn't got around to getting it, so I was thrilled when my parcel arrived in the mail. I had finally got the set through the kindness of wonderful friends.

As many women would experience, I was just so worried I would miscarry this pregnancy. I couldn't contemplate how I would cope. It seemed like it was a haze to push my thoughts into how I would deal with this if I had a miscarriage and I couldn't process it properly. I thought of many women before me who'd been through this and knowing how tough women are, they would carry on to the best of their ability. Would I end up being in this position? If I did, I would have to manage like many women before me who have experienced this. I tried to talk myself into accepting if a miscarriage were to happen, it was nature taking over and I couldn't stop this or even challenge it. I was helpless to this happening or not.

I tried to anticipate accepting the worst-case scenario as a mechanism to put up boundaries so I wouldn't replay the same worries over and over. Easier said than done, but I needed to take control and do something with these worrying thoughts. I learned this watching Doctor Phil. I learned through IVF to not project too many 'what if' thoughts as they may or may not eventuate. I invest my energy based on facts as the worry may never eventuate and if it did, I knew I would try to the best of my ability to deal with it. I know that each pregnancy had its own risks associated, and I was not free from that regardless of what I did to get this pregnancy. I was as vulnerable as any other pregnant woman. I was protecting my body and doing all I could to keep my nutrition and fluids adequate and rest as much as possible, and that's the extent of the control I had.

I was away for a weekend and was laying down and felt an obvious flutter from my lower stomach area. It was 12 November 09, and I was sixteen weeks pregnant. I'd just felt my baby move for the first time, which made me so happy. Another milestone locked in and each one that occurred from now on would just mean I was getting closer and closer to meeting my baby.

I arrived for my seventeen-week scan with my

Obstetrician, Dr Jyotica Ruba, knowing I would find out if I was having a boy or a girl. I decided early on there were so many moments where I had to wait for results through IVF that I didn't want to make myself wait for this news if I didn't have to. I knew either way, I would be so happy and I could think about how I would decorate the nursery and some sewing projects I had in mind. I had a feeling I would have a girl. This feeling had been mixed, but on the day I was leaning towards a girl. I laid on the bed and Dr Ruba placed gel on my stomach. I was about to experience another splendid moment in this miracle pregnancy. I will soon know what the gender of my baby will be.

When Dr Ruba conducted the ultrasound, I was watching her intently and listening to everything she said and did. Time seemed to freeze as it felt like it was taking so long. I kept still and couldn't speak and waited patiently, then I heard five very life changing and comforting words from a delighted obstetrician.

Dr Ruba said, "Jodi, you're having a boy."

Oh, wow a boy, how sweet. I love little boys, and I would have one of my own. I felt like I was on a euphoric high. The gender news was wonderful, and either way I knew I'd be happy, but it was also confirmation that all was travelling along well and my baby was safe (and alive). As I grew up with an older brother and younger sister, everything was pink when my sister was born. It would be a whole different experience with this little one and I just couldn't wait to get home and picture my whole house blue.

At my twenty-week scan, I was intently reading the sonographer to look for some signs from her that my baby was well. I could barely get a word out of the lady. She didn't seem like she was really interested in what she was doing, which was disappointing because I was bursting out of my skin to know if my baby looked okay. I remember feeling really deflated. It tainted the experience. After a number of images were obtained, I asked her did my baby look okay.

She said, "Yes, it does."

And that's the extent of the conversation during the whole ultrasound. I know Radiologists can't comment about the scan in medical terms, so I thanked her for her time when I left. One image was Jy holding his two fingers up, which represented the peace sign. I'm a simple, peaceful person and I found it to be such a beautiful image.

I secretly hoped to make it to the twenty-six-week mark heartbeat. I believed if my baby was born prematurely, it may have a chance of surviving with a lot of care and support from this point. I was at the shops and felt some tightness in my lower tummy and it didn't feel right. I went to the hospital and it turned out I had Braxton Hicks contractions. They sent me home with a safe report on my baby.

I only ever had enforced rests between IVF attempts. They were because my body needed to recover in between cycles, or because of the Christmas period, which meant I couldn't start again from early December onwards. This meant I would start again when cycles resumed again in January. Christmas was difficult for me because I didn't have my baby to celebrate with and it was the longest period of enforced rest I had. I still enjoyed my Christmas with my family and the joy the children in our family experienced on that day.

It was the Christmas of 2009 and I was on holidays at the Gold Coast, Queensland, Australia. It was special because it could be the only Christmas that I may be pregnant. The strain of those sad Christmas Days with no baby before was no longer to be. I sure knew this pregnancy was a blessing and not knowing what the future held, I didn't know if I would get pregnant again. I got a photo with Santa and declared that Jy's first Santa photo as my beautiful tummy was really showing by now. Santa asked me what I would like for Christmas and I said, "A delayed Christmas present in March please," and patted my tummy.

Santa winked at me and said, "I'll see what I can do."

On this holiday I had a 4D scan of my baby. They'd set the room up with a large screen on the front wall and reclining lounge chairs in front of the bed where I laid. Once Jy appeared on the screen we were amazed at the detail and the features we could see on my baby's face. I was just staring at the screen in astonishment. Jy decided he would remain asleep and didn't want to be part of this exciting adventure I'd looked forward to. The nurse tried a few techniques to wake Jy up and she asked me to get down on my hands and knees and crawl around the floor. Yes, I just did type that. I crawled around the floor to see if Jy would wake up. I only did this briefly as I felt that Jy wanted to sleep and a picture of him wasn't more important than him resting. I got up and said to the lady it doesn't matter, my baby wants to sleep so I will leave him be. I worried a little that maybe something was wrong with my baby as he didn't wake through all the activity. He woke soon after leaving the scan, so my worry faded away.

The pictures I received were so beautiful.

The nurse advised me they couldn't possibly charge me for a full package, which is what I'd ordered. She said as she couldn't take many photos because of my sleeping baby. As a result, she would only charge me for a gender scan. She again confirmed I was having a boy. The quality of the pictures and the detail they showed amazed me. I thought my baby had handsome features.

I then proceeded to my appointment to check if I had gestational diabetes, which I did. This startled me a little because I was concerned about what this meant for my baby. My holiday was due to end, and I returned home to an educational class about diabetes and how to manage the condition. I discovered I would need more needles as I couldn't manage my condition through diet alone. Arrrrrh, more needles! I couldn't seem to avoid them. I commenced counting the carbohydrates in every serve of food I had. It's actually quite a great way to eat as you eat regular meals throughout the day and in portion control sizes, which is to me the healthy way to eat.

Upon returning home from holidays, I commenced regular visits with my Endocrinologist, who assessed my eating plans of which I'd been documenting and advised the dosage of insulin accordingly. I was to inject four shots of insulin in my stomach every day for the remaining nine weeks of my pregnancy. I had an incident at home at around thirty-five weeks where my reading was just below two, which is low. I couldn't think clearly and knew my plan to save this situation was to have some jelly beans, so I did that to balance my levels back out and it worked. Thank goodness!

I received the most wonderful news. Amanda had given birth to twin boys from her last two frozen embryos one month before I was due to give birth to Jy. Prior to their implant, Amanda decided after many gruelling years, these two embryos were her last attempt. This makes me shiver. I still look at Amanda today with amazement. I'm so proud of her.

The good news just kept coming. Ian and Rosalie phoned me to advise they were having another baby and I would become an aunty again. I was absolutely delighted that Rosalie and I would be pregnant at the same time. I would then have someone close to share part of my pregnancy with, which was just wonderful.

I wanted to stay at work as long as I could because the possibility of passing out with the diabetes frightened me. Being home alone all day would mean no one would know if I fainted. Dr Ruba would be overseas and was due to return to work on a particular Monday, so we'd chosen the following Thursday as the elective caesarean delivery date. This would mean I was 38.5 weeks gestation upon giving birth. Dr Ruba wanted me to work until thirty-six weeks and rest for the remaining two-and-a-half weeks. As I was a high-risk pregnancy, she would deliver a little earlier than full term. I trusted her experience and went along with her plan.

At the thirty-six-week mark, when Dr Ruba was away, I felt well enough to work. As part of my routine check with my Endocrinologist, I asked if it would be possible to receive a certificate for work to state I could work until thirty-eight weeks. I explained my reasons of not wanting to be home alone should anything happen with my sugar levels. At work I would be surrounded by people and know they would call for help if I needed it. I was issued a certificate and planned to work another two weeks. My job wasn't physically strenuous, and I also knew the two weeks I worked would mean I could take an extra four weeks leave at half pay when my baby was actually here.

In the weeks leading up to finishing work, I bought

products for home in bulk, which were nappies and cleaning products. I tried to buy anything I could store at home and as a result would reduce my grocery bill each fortnight while I was on maternity leave. I planned to stay on maternity leave as long as financially possible as I wanted to enjoy this beautiful baby as long as I could before returning to work. I also didn't take it for granted this may be the only pregnancy and child I would have as who knows what the future holds, regardless of our desires. I planned to use my full pay annual leave and convert it to half pay so I could double the amount of time I would be on leave. To do this, I didn't use a lot of my annual leave during the years of IVF in the hope I could use it one day in addition to the maternity leave my employer provided. I also converted some of my long service leave to half pay and could then take twelve months' maternity leave in total.

I had a team of people at work who'd taken superb care of me during my pregnancy and they continued to do so until I worked my last day. They presented me with some beautiful gifts and there were a few tears as some people had worked with me throughout my entire IVF journey. I thanked my colleagues and managers for their support through what had been a difficult era in my life (IVF and losing my Dad). Yet it had also been wonderful with people being so happy for me as they watched my pregnant tummy grow.

When I walked out the doors of work on my last day, I believed I was about to embark on a journey that would change everything for me. It would change how I felt, and how I saw the world through a child's eyes. It was a milestone for me to be walking out of work to have a baby. To this point, I'd worked for nineteen years and dreamed about taking maternity leave to start my family. Well, the time had come and I could not wait for this journey to begin next week.

I was trying to get my gestational diabetes under control. My levels should have been between three and seven and they were fluctuating and I wasn't eating anything that I shouldn't be, so I headed into the diabetes clinic to get some guidance. I had come so far and would do whatever was needed to bring my baby home safely.

I had bought a newborn's baby suit and embroidered Jy's name and expected due date on the back. This would be the suit Jy would come home from the hospital in. On my first day of maternity leave, I had my final obstetrician appointment with Dr Ruba and showed her the suit. I politely requested we needed to deliver in three days on Thursday as the suit is embroidered already and I didn't want to unpick it. Dr Ruba laughed and said she will do her best to stick to the schedule.

I then went home and rested for the next two-and-a-half days as they would be the remaining days of my life without a child. I didn't want to overdo it or more so, risk anything in these final days of my pregnancy. I was nesting. It entered my mind about my baby not surviving these last few days. It was just the worry of something going wrong. The only way I could combat it was to let the thoughts pass through but be strong, to not let them stay long and hope for the best.

I can honestly say I did not take for granted one day of my pregnancy. No one knows if they will ever be pregnant again and I treated this pregnancy as if it was my last in case it was. I captured all the milestone moments and was grateful for every moment, even the sickness as it told me my baby was staying with me. Easier to type that now opposed to when you feel so ill.

The night before Jy's birth had a mystical feel in the air. It would be the last night of my life not being a parent. I had to this point grabbed life with both hands and made plenty of opportunities to enjoy most things I had wanted to do before I became a mother.

Because I'd prepared myself to be available in my mother role, I was content with the life I'd had before becoming a parent. I was ready for this next phase in my life. I ensured I'd packed my hospital bag and laid my clothes out for the next day. As I did every night of my pregnancy, I said good night to my child, only this time I added, "We will finally meet each other tomorrow." I had an early night to bank up some sleep in case I didn't sleep well or needed to top up for the following night, which would be my first night as a mother.

CHAPTER TWENTY-TWO

Ripping down the sheet

The day finally arrived. I was thirty-six years and three months old and today would rate as one of my best in history. Today I would meet my son. I would see what he looked like, what he smelled like, how soft his skin was and I knew I would stare into his eyes and melt away. I was feeling emotional and unsure how I would be when I gave birth, whether I would cry so many tears or not cry at all through amazement. Either way, I knew I would fulfil a long-held desire to become a mother today.

I was ecstatic, yet nervous when I woke. I felt like a child at Christmas time waiting to unwrap my presents. Throughout this IVF journey, I'd taught myself to leave my troubles or worries for another day when it was bedtime. I could at least reset in my sleep as it felt like it was the only place I didn't have to be strong. This wasn't easy to master and I certainly didn't perfect it, but I did help myself as much as I could with constructive thinking. I enjoyed a good sleep and felt I'd had enough rest when I woke. This made me feel strong to face the day. The worry for me was giving birth, even though I was having a planned caesarean. To say I was scared was an understatement. I'd no idea how I would do this. How would I handle a caesarean? I just hoped everything would be okay.

I'd eaten sensibly during my pregnancy and drank plenty of water. I wasn't aiming for any particular weight to end up at, I just made sure I ate properly. I got on the scales and gained 8kgs during my pregnancy. I took many photos on this morning prior to leaving home as it would be the last time I left my home as I knew it, particularly the nursery which was proudly set up. The pitter patter of a baby would soon fill this house with delight. I took lots of photos of my beautiful pregnant tummy which measured 110cms.

They expected me at the hospital at 9am for a mid-afternoon delivery. My hospital bag had been packed for a few weeks now. I couldn't think of anything else to add, so I grabbed my bag and made my way out the front. I noticed a beautiful red rose in my garden, which is one of my favourite flowers, and took a photo. I didn't notice this rose yesterday. A rose is resilient. It needs little to survive, but the more love you give a rosebush, the more beautiful it blossoms. I wanted to capture as much as I could about the day my baby arrived. I took a photo of the Ford Falcon car I went to hospital in as I imagined Jy saying how old the car was when he gets older. I also took a photo of the price of petrol at the petrol station, which was $1.24 per litre for unleaded. I stopped to buy the Daily Telegraph newspaper so Jy would know what happened on the day he was born. I planned to create a time capsule for Jy and all these items would tell a wonderful story.

The car ride to the hospital was a blur. I was lost in the wonder of what the day would bring. I arrived at the hospital and checked in. This was it. As I walked down the corridor in the maternity ward, I bumped into a man from work whose wife had their baby a few days prior. They were getting ready to go home. I tried to gauge how calm they were. That would be me in a few days, I just had to get through this afternoon. I congratulated my colleague and his wife and they wished me well. I made my way to my room and sat up on the bed and the nerves were off the scale. I'd been so worried I'd go into natural labour, something I'd been petrified of experiencing forever. I hadn't even read up on having a natural labour. I convinced myself the only way I could do this was through a caesarean.

I know women are built to bear children and give birth naturally, but throughout my adult life I just could not comprehend how my body would do it. More so, if I was trapped in the pain of a natural birth, how would I tolerate the pain? I know this has been going on since time began. But no matter how I convinced myself our bodies are made for this, and with medical intervention and pain relief, I just could not process it. I was absolutely petrified of giving birth and was shaking in my boots. I decided to have the caesarean when they mentioned this would be the safest way to get the baby out because of my gestational diabetes. Every decision I have made so far was to bring a child into the world, so after they explained their reasoning, I was sold this was the way for me and my baby. I sighed in relief I wouldn't have to face a huge fear of mine, a natural birth.

I admire women who've had a natural birth because that hasn't been my experience and I can't relate to that. My hat goes off to you and your courage for doing something I thought I couldn't. Do I feel I have missed out? No, not at all. It's ironic a lady like me who fought so hard to get a baby was so petrified of how it would be born. I thought all along I would just deal with that on the day. Well, today is that day and I'm freaking out.

I sat in the room and felt my baby hiccup in my stomach. This is something I'd enjoyed towards the end of my pregnancy. I shed a few tears, and they connected to the deepest part of my heart. I'd longed for this moment in time for most of my adult life. I knew I was meant to be a mum. This was the moment I'd taken a pounding physically, financially and emotionally to arrive at. I do not know how I did it. I was waiting to be called in to deliver my baby and I was so petrified. I knew there was no point holding back any tears and I would burst into tears the moment I heard this precious little person. I talked to my baby and said to please stick with me and let's do this safely. We'd been a great team so far and had one last significant step to take together. I pretended I was wrapping layers of protection around both of us and the doctors who would bring this miracle to life on the outside.

I'm crying while typing this book now. It's still so raw. I completed ten unsuccessful rounds of IVF and this precious boy who is lying beside me sleeping peacefully as I type is what it was all for. I love him with all my heart. Goodness knows how I'll be typing about the moment he was born!

I changed into the robe and the nurse came in to give me instructions and advised it would be about mid-afternoon, depending on whether any emergencies arrived. My wonderful mother was with me and she'd always been my rock. I spoke to Mum about how I would handle going into natural labour if it were to happen now, before the scheduled caesarean. Mum said we are built to do this and if I had to, she knew I would just take it in my stride and do what needed to be done. I said, "Mum, I haven't read up on anything." (I'm laughing now. Trust me to take such a punt.).

She said, "You will be fine, love. You're in the right place," and nodded her reassurance.

This settled me down and we guessed what time we thought Jy would be born. Mum said 3.43pm, and I said 3.08pm.

The wardsmen arrived in my doorway, and I took a huge deep breath. This is it. They'll wheel me away and I will come back through these doors holding my baby. They wheeled me into a waiting bay and I felt helpless and frightened and wondered how this would end up. I replaced this worry with trust as I'd replaced sadness with hope during my IVF attempts. I'd trusted Dr Ruba every step of the way and I leaned into the thought of her experience and knowledge pulling us through.

I felt like I was juggling a ball of fear into the air, catching it and throwing up another of pure elation. I had a photo taken of me at this point. I had my blue hair cap on and I was lying on the bed outside the theatre and you can see the look of fear in my eyes. I was on the extreme cusp of emotions and it captures how frightened and happy I was at this moment.

They advised me to walk into the theatre and I noticed the bed and the special machines and equipment in the room. A male doctor instructed me on what would happen with the epidural. I've explained how much I don't like needles, well this one would have to top the list of needles that terrified me. Right about now, I was thinking maybe I would have dodged having this needle if I had a natural birth, but I was immediately satisfied I'd chosen this path. He advised me to sit still. I was to sit on the bed facing away from the doctor and he would numb the lower part of my back. Then I would feel a small sting. Well, when you are asked to do something in the nervous state I was in, I worried I would shake even more. I just wanted the moment to be over. I didn't want to brace myself to be still any longer. I didn't share my fear with the doctor as I didn't want him to concentrate on anything other than giving me the epidural correctly. I was so worried I wouldn't be able to hold still for too long. Thankfully, I focused and stayed still.

My super star Obstetrician, Dr Ruba, appeared like a protective angel. She reassured me that she would take good care of my baby and I. Dr Ruba handled my nerves spectacularly throughout our pregnancy consultations and she just knew how to settle me down. It was such a relief to see her and know she hadn't been caught in traffic! Her presence, confidence and professionalism allowed me to slightly relax!

Dr Ruba introduced her colleague, who was a male obstetrician. He introduced himself and said he was aware of my story to get this baby and said it was an honour to be part of this delivery. I said, "Oh really, thank you. It's lovely to meet you and thank you for your assistance today." I was flattered he'd heard of me and knew my story. To me, I was just Jodi Maher, who had a difficult time getting pregnant. To him, this is why people go into medicine, to help and see the impossible become possible.

It's about this time the camera started rolling from my side of the blue sheet. I wanted to film this amazing experience. I wanted to do this because when

I'm emotional; I miss recalling events and thoughts and I didn't want to miss a moment here. This would allow me time later to reflect on the whole magical experience. As a woman and very soon, a new mother, I anticipated I may not be able to express in words a true reflection of the love I knew I'd feel for this precious soul. I wanted to be able to reflect and watch this incredible achievement over and over again. As a result, I have this moment captured on film. I also wanted to show my son, later on in his life, the moment he was born.

Machines continue to beep and I could hear suction noises. I'd cried out all the sad tears and only the happy tears remained. There were years' worth of tears I'd built up and reserved for this moment in time. They'd been parked away in a bubble of hope. They were ready to fall. The bubble was bursting. I couldn't stop the tears. I didn't want to stop tears. I could feel the lump in my throat. I felt the release of many years of being strong, against all odds, was about to leave me. I would feel free. My yearning mummy heart was about to be rewarded.

My time had come. This is it. The wait was almost over.

I shared part of my transcript in the first chapter. Here's what happened next.

Baby: Crying (from the other side of the sheet). Let me hold my son! 4.52 pm and I've just heard the most wonderful sound. I heard my child. Yes, my child. The wait was over. I was elated. I was proud. I exhaled and said to myself, "We did it!." I just heard my child! In this second, my son was communicating with me, his mummy. He was crying because they'd taken him from his comfort, me, the safe place he was used to and entered a whole new world. He didn't realise that Mummy was right here waiting for him.

Me: My tear bubble exploded. Within one second of hearing Jy's cry, I obliviously, and contrary to medical procedure/advice, ripped down the blue sheet of the operating theatre after hearing my son for the first time. I could not see him. It did not matter what he looked like; but I needed to see him to believe that he was there. As I was still gripping a tissue in my left hand from the finger prick earlier, the pole dislodged from the sheet and crashed to the ground with an almighty bang! Within two seconds of Jy being born, I'd made a loud ruckus! It wasn't New Year's Eve, but I sure made the theatre sounded like fireworks. My baby was being held in the air surrounded by a loud bang thanks to his mumma. The sheet was still erected on one side and I could only lift my head slightly off the pillow and then I glimpsed part of my child's head. I could see black hair, but I could not see anything else. I was yearning to see his face, his body, I wanted to count his fingers and toes. I wanted to touch his skin and smell him. I felt my body, well the part of it I could feel, just melt and I continued to cry. My heart was racing.

Male doctor: "Oh, don't reach over the top… sorry."

Obstetricians: "Oh, ah."

Dr Ruba: "Ohhhhhh… Happy Birthday. Ohhhhh… This is your little one," she said as she held Jy in the air towards my direction with happy and excited eyes behind her mask.

The wait was over. I couldn't believe I was in this very moment. It felt like a magical dream.

My baby was being held in the air with one hand each supporting my baby's bottom and head, while being positioned at the right height, within my full view, which allowed me to see all of my miracle for the very first time. What a breathtaking moment it was. I witnessed a miracle being held in the air before me.

My baby had both arms opened wide and the theatre light above highlighted dark hair and the most delicate angelic features on a beautiful little face. I scanned my baby's body and determined my precious baby was a boy (Dr Ruba had got it correct at the 17 week scan.) He was perfect and most of all, he was all I imagined, dreamed and hoped for him to be and more. He was real and he was my son.

I was mesmerised at the divine sight before me and I felt winded with overwhelming excitement and believing this moment was real. I had butterflies and my heart was racing with excitement and then, I heard the most incredible sound.

My baby let out another cry that was deep, consistent and extremely loud to let the world know he had arrived. (I'm still crying, then and as I type now.)

Male obstetrician: Clamping and cutting the cord.

Me: crying. I felt like I sunk into the bed and cried and couldn't stop. I exhaled and breathed out relief. I closed my eyes and pictured Jy being lifted before me again and this vision will never leave my memory.

Dr Ruba immediately handed Jy to the paediatrician.

They took him from my view and I couldn't believe it. I was so emotionally overwhelmed. I just could not stop crying. I'd pictured this moment for many years and all I could do was continue to hope I would be fortunate enough to feel it one day and bring a life into the world. Well, I just did that! It really was a defining moment in my life. My heart felt full of pride and was bursting with love for this precious little person who I would cherish forever. I was also proud of myself. I'd been rewarded with this beautiful gift, my child who'd just made me a mother for the first time and what an instantaneous, unconditional miracle bond we formed together. A bond that would stand the test of time.

All I yearned for now was to hold him, to touch him, to smell him, to feel his skin, to introduce myself as his mummy. Now I had to wait and this wait was the happiest throughout the whole journey. I took in all the sounds in the room, including the cry of my son and what a sweet sound it was. Each breath he took made me feel more settled his lungs were working properly. I would have to wait for the clearance Jy was okay before I could see him again.

My son cried again and through my flood of tears, his delicate cry sent shivers up my neck and the happiness I felt in this moment was one of my favourite moments in time.

I am still crying writing this chapter as I did the moment I heard my baby for the first time in the delivery room. I was yearning to hear more crying, and I thought please give me a really big loud cry, my baby, and he responded and opened his lungs. The comfort that sound gave me was what I'd yearned for all my adult life. My son was alive, he was safe, and he was finally here! The part of my body I could feel, which was from my arm pits up to my head was feeling free and relieved and I cried and cried and I just couldn't stop. I could feel the tears coming right from my heart. The part of me that had constantly backed up for so long was being freed. I let out years of pain in these tears. A dream had just come true. I could feel the anguish leave me in an instant and it was replaced by feeling empowered, proud, happy and content because any second I would hold my baby for the first time.

Male doctor: Well done, now let's pop that back up (referring to the sheet). He certainly looks and sounds pretty good so I don't think he'll be away for too long," as the camera returns to me.

Jy: Crying (over at the trolley getting checked by the paediatrician and nurse).

Me: Crying (unable to speak).

Jy: Crying really loud!

Me: I had a moment where, despite being temporarily paralysed, I felt the desire to get up and get him. My mother instincts kicked in and Jy had only been born for a few minutes. At this point, I felt the force of a mother's love for their child. I wondered whether being in a new environment frightened him and I hoped his cry didn't mean he was scared because I heard him stop and then start again. I knew he was just settling and everything was new for him too, but I knew he needed his mummy as much as I needed him. Bring my boy to me now! I found comfort in overhearing the paediatrician and nurse talking and they seemed happy with everything and I knew he'd be back with me soon.

Me: Crying (still unable to speak, tears rolling down my cheeks).

Male doctor: "Well done, let's pop that off now. The oxygen is just for the baby." (Removing oxygen mask from me.)

Me: Crying a deep sob of uncontrollable happy tears.

The relief in this moment was amazing. By this time, I'd two minutes to briefly process what just happened and my eyes were closed and I was still crying from a deep down place, right down in the deepest chamber of my heart. We connect these tears to feelings we bury or don't visit often and when they come out, they are so powerful and moving, like I cried when Dad and Nan passed away. These powerful tears in that moment came from that place, but they were tears of sheer joy, delight and success yet I was so calm in my thoughts and was uncharacteristically so quiet. It was an internal realisation of what I'd just achieved. "My son, we did it my love, we did it, we made it," was all I could think at this point.

Baby: Still crying (as the camera moved towards him).

Nurse: "He is model material," (as she wiped my baby). I didn't realise she said this until I watched the video later.

Baby: crying from deep down. (You can see his chest inhaling and exhaling on the video as he took big breaths.) The nurse was talking to my son and said to him that she was wrapping him up to take him over to meet his mummy. The video is pointing in my direction and the magical moment she hands me my son is forever etched in my mind.

My son was placed on my chest, and my chin was quivering from crying. His eyes were closed, and he still had vernix caseosa over his face which protected Jy's skin from the constant exposure to the amniotic fluid in the womb. He was making a murmuring sound. Despite feeling and knowing him for the past nine months, this was the first time I could touch my son in the flesh.

I supported the bottom half of Jy with my right hand which was taped with cords and the IV drip. My left hand stroked my son's face for the first time and the feel of his soft skin made my mummy heart explode like a firecracker lighting up the sky. The tears were rolling down my cheeks. I'd dreamed of this moment through such heartache and here I was, holding my son. I said, "Hello my Jy, I'm your mummy and I love you with all of my heart," and I whispered to Jy, "thank you."

In that moment, I touched my son and I put my other hand on my mouth in awe and shock and I felt happiness rush through me. I continued to break down crying tears of happiness. Jy was trying to open his left eye to see me and hear the voice he knew so well. I watched intently as he partially opened his eyelid and I got a glimpse of his eye and I melted. We just laid eyes on each other for the first time and I couldn't believe this moment was real.

Jy opened up a part of me I didn't know was there. I fell in love in a crazy mother kind of way in that moment. He was still making noises, and I watched him move his mouth. I instinctively and gently rubbed and pat his bottom to soothe him as only mothers know how to do. My chest felt free. I felt like the heavy load I'd been carrying for years was now being replaced with the weight of a baby on my chest and I just couldn't believe how lucky I was.

I then worried about the grunting noises Jy was making. I thought something was wrong and the pit of my stomach felt sick.

The nurse came over and said, "What's are these noises for, little one?"

She seemed to walk away, not worried. I asked was he okay, and the doctor said that he was, and I hoped they knew what they were doing. (Of course, they did.) I now realised my concern for my child had only just begun. Once I settled back down, I had the most beautiful photo taken of Jy and me and the relief in my eyes says it all. "I'm a mum now. Look at my son!"

I did cry a tear for my Dad. He would have been so proud of me. He knew how difficult achieving one pregnancy was for me. I was holding his grandson and that made me feel very proud of myself for doing everything within my power to be in that moment. I'm sure he was smiling at Jy and me from above and was probably doing a little victory dance!.

They took Jy to the nursery for monitoring and me to recovery. It wasn't long before they reunited us and I enjoyed a relaxing cuddle with him back in my room. I spent the next few hours admiring my child and bonding with him. I was watching him and taking in all his sounds and his smell. It was time to put him to sleep for the night and I slipped into my new mother role so well. I fed him and wrapped him and watched him fall to sleep. I was so proud and honoured to be this little boy's mother. I felt so blessed.

I reflected on the proudest day of my life. I don't even remember ripping the sheet down or the doctor asking me not to reach over the top. I discovered this when I watched the video for the first time and I can't believe I did it. I can from my inquisitive side. Jy was born and I couldn't see him and even though my body was disconnected from my arms and hands, I still felt something. My instincts kicked in and I wanted to see my baby.

I must admit giving birth is something that's petrified me my entire adult life. But my experience was so beautiful. Wonderful doctors and nurses supported me and I faced my fear of needles head on. No matter which way I turned, I wasn't getting away from them unless I relented on having a baby and that wouldn't happen while I'd the strength to keep going. The epidural was beyond my realm of comprehension because I was so frightened of this. I worried I might not make it or it could cause me a long-term injury or my son might not pull through the birth. Giving birth was my biggest fear in life and I felt the fear and did it anyway. I conquered one of my biggest personal challenges and I was so proud of myself.

As I listened to my baby's breathing as he slept peacefully beside me, I still couldn't feel the lower half of my body from my birth. What I did feel was the pressure release from my mind. I took a moment to reflect on the whole IVF journey and in particular that day. It felt like a three and a half year pregnancy with all the IVF attempts and the actual pregnancy itself. I'd protected my body for years as though I was pregnant to keep myself in optimum condition.

This pregnancy phase had come to a sweet end. I looked down at my stomach which had reduced in size and looked over to my son. I cried. I was so proud of what I'd achieved and what I fought for. I was so proud that through some trying moments, I kept going and brought this beautiful child into the world safely.

I'd said good night to my baby in my stomach every night since 11 July 2009 when I found out I was pregnant. I'd only ever dreamed about this moment, but tonight was different. Tonight, I said goodnight to my beautiful bundle of joy, sleeping peacefully in the hospital bassinette beside me. I had a big proud smile on my face and kissed his forehead and held his hand. His tiny fingers could barely wrap around my finger.

I was thirty-six years old, and I finally was blessed with a precious child. The planets finally aligned, and I was absolutely delighted. I was more tired and lethargic than I've ever been, but I couldn't fall off to sleep. I was too excited and kept looking at my baby in amazement and trying to work out if I was in a dream. It was a beautiful moment when I leaned over and touched my son again. A tear of joy rolled down my cheek.

Life couldn't get any sweeter than the day my precious child was born.

CHAPTER TWENTY-THREE

The Next Five Years

I left hospital following Jy's birth with a smile on my face and a deliriously happy mummy heart. I took photos throughout the whole journey of leaving the hospital to our arrival at Jy's new house. I arrived home and felt complete. I'd wanted this precious child for so long and I felt so content.

I am a person who loves my sleep, and I found it a whole new world waking up every few hours, but I had an adrenalin rush and an adorable child to care for. I had moments where I could see my whole life had changed and it would never be the same. I had this little dependent child who was relying on me and while it was a little daunting, I instinctively knew what to do. I was so proud of myself and my son as we had both slipped into a great routine and were happy and healthy. I filmed each event in which Jy had his firsts;

his smile, his bath at home, him yawning and was in amazement that this miracle was in my arms and heart every day.

For the first month of Jy's life, I'd been waking him for feeds every three hours. I don't know if this was acceptable in the eyes of the professionals, but I was so worried about a little baby being able to wake themselves if something was wrong with them. The assumption he would wake himself kept me awake, so I started setting my alarm. It was Good Friday 2010, four weeks after Jy was born. My alarm clock went off at 3am and I picked Jy up out of his bassinette and he was lethargic. I tried to feed Jy but I could tell something wasn't right. I was immediately worried and I gently put some water on his face to try to get a reaction. I don't know if in hindsight this was the right thing to do. I got a response, but I knew I needed to get to the hospital as Jy was limp like a rag doll.

I drove straight to the hospital and was taken through the emergency department immediately. Someone took us to a holding bay. They assessed Jy and moved us into a room which read 'Resuscitation' on the door. Why are we going in here? Is Jy going to die? I remember thinking this wasn't a good sign. Please, don't take my son away from me. I panicked and convinced myself to this point that Jy will be okay, but now I worried. I could read the doctors and knew they were worried. I hoped they would find out what was wrong and quickly. I stood by the bed as they hooked Jy up to machines. I cried. A pulse and a heartbeat showed on the screen and I breathed a sigh of relief. I was grateful for this moment. I felt Jy had a chance.

However, I still didn't know what was wrong or if he would make it or was hours, minutes or seconds from passing away. His eyes wouldn't open and he was skinny. I had a quiet word to my dad, who had passed away twenty-one months before. I said if Jy had to be taken from me now, to please look after him as I tried so hard to get him and I've only had him for four weeks. I was giving myself a chance to be prepared, and it was gut-wrenching. I never got the chance to say goodbye to Dad when he passed away. If my boy was leaving me, I wanted to have a chance this time to say goodbye to a precious loved one in the flesh.

I knelt beside my boy and his arms and legs were flopped out beside him and he had a bag over his groin area to catch a urine sample. I spoke quietly so no one in the room could hear me. It was roughly 4am in the still of the night and I said, "Jy, I love you, you can come through this my little man. You are strong, we are strong together, we are in the right place, just hold on. But if it's too tough for you and you can't fight it, please let go my son, be free from pain. Poppy will look after you and I will always love you."

He lay lifeless, but my hopes lay in the monitor which my eyes were glued to. There was a pulse and a heartbeat and this meant my boy was still alive. I needed to give Jy permission and I think I was also letting myself accept whatever may be, whatever I didn't have control over and hope that the doctors would help pull my baby through. It was a horrible moment to be in but I knew I needed to rise above somehow and give myself permission to be present, just in case I was moments away from losing Jy.

Many years later on 24 May 2014, I watched my mother lie beside her dying mother and Mum spoke to Nan in the same manner I had to Jy. Mum was giving Nan permission to go in case that is what Nan needed to hear. I thought how selfless it was of my mum to do that. I remember looking at my mum as she was talking to Nan, and I was in awe of Mum's selflessness and strength. I always admired my mum's softness, but this was just a whole new side of my mum I hadn't seen before. I fell in love, as only a daughter can, with my beautiful mother all over again in that moment. There were two women before me, my nan and my mum who were pioneers of strength and led our family proudly over the decades. It was terribly sad to watch through my falling tears, but it was a tender moment between a mother and daughter and was a blessing to witness this show of love. I didn't get this chance to be with Dad when he passed and I would have loved to have been with him, so I was pleased my mum was with her mum. I then remembered I had that similar chat with Jy on the resuscitation table and I knew exactly why Mum was saying what she was saying. Nan passed away within half hour surrounded by loving family.

Life is so precious.

A few hours passed, and I'd been nervously watching Jy for some progress and he opened his eyes, much to my delight. Another glimmer of hope! The scales were tipping in our favour and I experienced a rush of happiness underneath the worry. I stood up immediately to let Jy see me. I wanted him to feel someone familiar in the unfamiliar surroundings. I said hello out loud so he could also hear my voice. I asked him to be brave and we will work out what needs to happen to make him feel better.

After Jy stabilised, they moved us to a high

dependency room within the children's ward. It was a room where only one patient could be cared for. This was to ensure contamination was at a minimum and one-on-one care was available around the clock.

The team of resuscitation doctors decided Jy needed a lumbar puncture. This would tap the fluid from his brain to check for the more serious viruses like meningococcal and meningitis. I was worried at this point. My four-week old baby would have a needle in his back. They gave us a care flight teddy bear, and I had a photo taken with Jy and the bear at this moment. The look in my eyes is relief that Jy was in my arms, but I was exhausted. Jy nestled in my chest. I didn't know what lay ahead.

Jy had the lumbar puncture, and the results confirmed there were no serious viruses. What a relief. They placed Jy on antibiotics via a drip and I was grateful for the Ronald McDonald House down the hallway from Jy which gave me somewhere to collapse when I couldn't keep going. What a brilliant facility. I had a photo of Jy right near Ronald McDonald to show Jy when he is older how small he was. It was a place to have a shower and a sleep.

One doctor told me twenty-four hours later

after treating Jy in the resuscitation table they were concerned and I said I could read them and knew they were too. They tested Jy for the top six severe viruses and the conclusion was an unidentified virus. I was pleased to be walking out the doors with my son and heading home on day six. I became stricter on who could come near Jy and hold him as I'd no idea how he'd contracted this virus. I asked anyone who came to our house to wear a mask as I was petrified of having to relive this moment of sickness with Jy.

Jy was travelling along splendidly. He was smiling, and he was happy and was feeding well. I was adapting to life as a mother and it was tiring, but it was pure bliss. I was fortunate to spend time away from work and focus solely on my son. It was one of the most wonderful chapters of my life. I'd saved up all my leave at work and I was enjoying this precious time with Jy.

I took a close-up photo of Jy's face as he was asleep in his car seat. I showed Mum how gorgeous the photo was of Jy and Mum pointed out it was the exact profile of Jy taken during the 4D scan when I was still pregnant. The likeness is uncanny and I know that seems obvious as it's Jy in the same photo but the clarity between two photos, one inside my stomach and the other is astounding.

When Jy was six months old, we were briefly away from home and staying in a cabin at Scarborough, Queensland, Australia. Jy had a temperature that I wanted checked, so we went up to Redcliffe hospital. Little did we know we would leave this hospital with a nurse escorting us back home to Canberra on a plane with an oxygen tank.

They checked Jy's temperature and discovered Jy had a low oxygen reading when he slept. The bottom of Jy's neck looked like it was sinking in as he took in a breath. The doctors referred to it as a tracheal tug and fitted Jy with nose prongs. They connected him to oxygen when he slept. Teams of doctors would monitor Jy on their daily visit and decided to keep Jy on the oxygen to get his levels to an acceptable range. I was extremely tired, as I didn't know why this was happening to my boy and I was having trouble sleeping in the hospital. But as any parent would know who has a child in hospital, our tiredness becomes secondary to our desire to push through to nurse our child to better health.

I remember thinking at one stage and was wondering how I would get through today. I was just exhausted. I decided to get outside of the hospital walls and go for a walk outside with Jy. So, I put him in his pram and sat him upright so he could enjoy this adventure. I placed the portable oxygen tank that was kindly provided by the nursing staff under the pram. I hooked Jy up and off we went. We sat outside the hospital and I showed Jy the leaves that were blowing in the wind and was listening to his baby talk through the noise coming from his nose prongs. I was grateful for the hospital facilities, the nursing staff, the support we received and this precious bundle of joy who entered my life six months ago. I really was one lucky lady.

This little adventure went on for many days to break the time in hospital. Jy's oxygen statistics weren't improving. We trialled giving him no oxygen as he slept to compare it to the last reading, but the doctor decided Jy should remain on oxygen until his levels increased and stabilised. The issue was, we didn't know when this would be and we were over 1000 kilometres from home and our booked accommodation had now expired. I didn't have anywhere to stay, not that it looked like we would be released from hospital anytime soon. Jy could not sleep without oxygen and he was having naps during the day and his night sleep.

After discussions with the doctors, they decided we needed to get home somehow. They decided we would fly home; however it was a requirement that a nurse escort Jy and I on the plane as he was still a patient. And as we had to be connected to oxygen, it was a requirement by the doctors for the care and safety of their patient. So, on day nine, we boarded the plane bound for the next hospital. Jy fell asleep in the air on my lap and we turned the oxygen on. The plane ride was smooth, and I enjoyed flying, so it was a real highlight for me to be up in the air again. I didn't know how long we would be in the next hospital, but we arrived in Canberra with a waiting bed at the hospital. The nurse disconnected Jy from the portable oxygen and I thanked her for her care and wished her a safe journey back to Queensland. They hooked Jy up to the hospital oxygen next time he fell asleep, and the nurse watched over Jy while I showered. It was a long day. We were in a room with three other children and families and it was difficult to rest, but the main thing was Jy was where he needed to be and we were now only five minutes from home.

The paediatrician who monitored us was wonderful. Each day passed, and we checked for progress, but Jy was not improving. His levels declined as soon as he fell asleep. Many days had now passed, and I wondered how long we would have to stay for. My child wasn't well, and I looked around and knew other families were worried about their children who were sick. I wandered pass the high dependency unit that Jy was in when he was four weeks old and was so blessed that my son was cared for so diligently. Some staff remembered us from that visit and were doting over Jy. One lady said she will never forget Jy as she was in the room when he got his lumbar puncture at four weeks old. It's a grounding place to be in hospital because while your child is sick and it's the biggest worry you are facing, you know there have been some sad and happy stories inside those walls.

On day seventeen of being in hospital, the paediatrician indicated we could consider going home with an at home oxygen tank program. This option delighted me. The program involved Jy having the nose prongs connected day and night, and any time Jy slept I was to turn the oxygen machine on. I was to return to hospital with Jy once a week for him to have a sleep in hospital and be assessed by the paediatrician. This sounded like a plan I could manage. So, on day eighteen, we packed our bags and left hospital and an oxygen tank was delivered to our home (before his next sleep).

I was pleased to be home. I missed the comforts of home. I wanted to sleep in my own bed. Jy slept in the same room as me as I was uncomfortable at the thought of a six-month-old with prongs in his nose and cords attached sleeping away from me. I didn't have any nurses overseeing him, so I had to go forward with a plan I was comfortable with and made Jy safe. I was not willing to risk Jy rolling over with cords attached to him. I figured if there were self-settling issues later, I'd deal with them then. My aim was to keep Jy safe and alive.

I spent the remainder of my twelve months maternity leave taking Jy for weekly, then fortnightly sleep studies at the hospital as his oxygen levels stabilised.

Ian and Rosalie called to announce they'd delivered an adorable baby boy named Wyatt. He would be my precious nephew and along with his much older brother Allan (named after my dear dad), who is similar in age to David. I have a special connection with both these boys and I know I would feel forever blessed to have two beautiful nephews on Earth. They bring me so much joy and I'm so incredibly lucky to be their aunty. They absolutely adore Jy.

I was having separation worries from Jy as it was leading up to him going into child care so I could return to work. I was losing sleep and so worried about being away from my boy. I wanted to stay home with him permanently, but just couldn't manage that and keep everything else going financially. I surrendered to the awful feeling by thinking about how Jy would be exposed to other children and different activities. I gave him a big hug, left him at the child care centre and drove to work with many tears rolling down my cheeks. He was safe and with a good centre, so I knew I needed to move into the next phase of being a working mum.

They could monitor his medical condition at the day care centre, which brought me comfort. Jy made slow progress and was finally given clearance from post bronchiolitis obliterans (an uncommon and severe form of chronic obstructive lung disease in children that results from an insult to the lower respiratory tract) at eighteen months old.

Doctors advised Renée she was likely to require IVF to conceive her child when Jy was eighteen months old. Although Renée wasn't ready to have children at that point, I let Renée know I would be her surrogate if it ever got to that point for her. I was ten years older than Renée, but I'd just proven I could carry a child. I thought it may give Renée an option she could tuck away to use should she ever need to. From my side, doing another round would have just been that. It would have been a vehicle to carry a child. I was thrilled with not going through IVF anymore but would have easily signed up for round twelve to give my sister a chance to become a mother.

I loved our first Christmas together. I dressed Jy up as an elf and gave him a set of drums. We banged them and made lots of noise together. I always look for Christmas decorations with Joy on them, because that is Jy's name without the O. I cover the O with a picture of Jy and he has his own Christmas decorations.

I absolutely adored taking Jy for swimming lessons. Prior to his first lesson, I searched the internet for tips on how to teach children to swim. I learned that pouring water over Jy's head in the bath would get him used to the water. We lived in a cold climate, but the heated pool made it much easier to enjoy the swimming lesson. For over twelve months, I got into the pool with Jy to enjoy his lessons with him as he was young and I looked forward to taking Jy every week. Jy's star sign is a Pisces, and the symbol is a fish, which certainly is my boy who just loves swimming.

Over the next few years, I took many photos and videos of Jy to document each milestone and I recently looked back over those photos and the time just flies.

He has grown into a wonderful, well-mannered boy.

I was as emotional as any other parent on their child's first day of school. I was still in shock I had this precious child still after all these years. Jy was posing for photos for his first day of school but would not take one without his eyes crossed; it was his latest fad at the time. So, all his photos are of him being cheeky, despite my best attempts to get a photo with his eyes straight. We assembled at school and walked to Jy's classroom and I felt some tears roll down my cheek. My miracle was starting school and I couldn't have been prouder.

In the year our IVF children were in kindergarten, Amanda and I went to a seminar at work together. Afterwards, we got talking about IVF and how hard it was and it brought a tear to both our eyes. We both agreed the process changed us forever. It's who we became through the sheer heartache which created a whole new part of us.

A part I know recovered, but a scar most certainly remains. A scar means we took on something stronger than us and beat it.

CHAPTER TWENTY-FOUR

A Ring and a Flower for Mummy

From three years of age, I taught Jy to do three nice things for me every day. The idea was to instil the gift of giving from a young age and to teach him how to show love to his special people without spending money. I encouraged Jy to choose what nice things he could do for me and he decided they would be a kiss, a cuddle, and to pick me a flower. As Jy celebrates a new birthday, he gives me another flower when he collects them because everything in his world is about how old he is. I often watch Jy in a park and know he has stopped to choose a flower for me. I have found flowers in Jy's pockets and know he's picked them during the day at school and kept it for me. I took a photo of Jy hiding a flower behind his back and presenting it to one happy mummy. It is one of my favourite photos and memorable moments.

When Jy started kindergarten, I asked him what was the best thing about his day.

He said, "You picking me up from school."

Bless him! In his second week of school, Jy said he wanted to go to the shops, and I asked him what it was he needed. He responded with the most beautiful request. He said he wanted to take me to the shops to buy me a ring. I melted at the same time as feeling something special about this child, his sweetness, his desire to want to give to his mummy.

I asked Jy if he had any money to buy the ring and he checked his pockets and asked if I could take him home so he could get his coins. I explained it's nice to do things for people and as this was a special occasion, I asked if he would like me to add any extra money, if the ring cost more than his coins.

He said, "Yes please, Mummy, I like."

We went straight to the shops and fortunately there were many choices as it was near Valentine's Day. The shop assistant asked if she could help us and Jy said he wanted to buy a ring for his mummy. The lady thought it was a wonderful gesture and acknowledged Jy for being so precious. If only she knew just how precious this boy was.

As soon as Jy saw the ring with a heart, he said, "That's the one I want Mummy."

Jy picked out a beautiful pink heart-shaped dress ring with two diamonds on the side and I was delighted to have received such a beautiful gift from my son. This has become my favourite piece of jewellery and one I wear with pride and will treasure. It really symbolises this journey. Sharp point at the bottom of the heart (needles), curved edges of the heart (my pregnancy tummy), sparkly (the pregnancy phone call, watching my baby grow and the birth) and the two diamonds (a mother and son united by determination, love and hope).

I cried many tears and endured so, so much. Little did I know the day King of Pop passed away was the beginning for us. I am continuing my family's tradition of raising Jy with music and living each day enjoying the sweetest sound of all, my child.

CHAPTER TWENTY-FIVE

My Jy's Adorable Comments

I kept a record of Jy's comments and stories from his first couple of years of school. They are as follows:

1. As I was walking Jy to school, he said, "Some days I will be a grown up, some days I will be a giant, some days I'll be a big person."

2. When Jy was four, he said, "Mummy, I just want to be five."

3. I overheard Jy whispering to his toy car in bed, he was saying "I love you Roary. You are the best car ever and I won't let you down."

4. Jy asked me why people had fur (hair) on their

legs.

5. Jy gave me a biscuit and said, "That's what friends do."

6. I was wearing a blue shirt and Jy said, "Blue is my favourite colour and blonde is my favourite hair."

7. Jy was learning to count to 100, and he said, "Mum are you 40?" I replied, "Yes Jy." Jy said, "That's nearly 100 Mum!" And I smiled and said, "Yes, Jy, you are getting good at counting!"

8. Jy asked if we could go to Nanny's country next week, referring to Nanny Cheryl (my Mum) as she lived in a different state.

9. "Where did you get me from Mummy? From the shops?". I responded, "No, you grew in my tummy." Jy then asked if he was a tiny baby like a mouse. I said he was tiny like a jelly bean when he first started to grow in my tummy. He then asked how he came out of my tummy and I explained the doctors helped to get him out. Jy said, "Wow!"

10. Jy was most upset he'd left his guitar at preschool and at bedtime asked through tears if we could go to

the day care centre to get his guitar as it will be lonely. I explained the guitar will be playing songs for all the other toys and that we can get it tomorrow. Jy settled and said, "Okay, Mummy."

11. "If you swallow me, Mummy, then you'll have another Jy."

12. Jy was in the back seat of the car as I was driving and he commented on the 110 kilometre per hour street sign. He asked, "Mum are you doing 110?" as he looked at the speedometer and I said, "Yes." He asked, "Can you do 220?" and I said, "I'm not allowed to drive that fast Jy. The police will pull me over and give me a ticket. I have to drive no faster than the sign posted limit of 110." He said, "Oh, okay, Mummy. I don't want you to go to jail."

13. I picked Jy up from school and was going to drive into our driveway when Jy asked if I could keep driving. He said, "We have moved to a new house and I'll show you how to get there." So I agreed. I followed Jy's instructions, which led us to our local grocery store. I asked if this was our new house and he said, "No, Mum, I tricked you. I would like a chocolate egg please." So, I enjoyed the humour of the moment and walked into the grocery store and bought Jy his

favourite egg.

14. "You are the best mumma I've ever seen."

15. "You are the best mum ever, ever, ever, ever, ever, ever. That's how much I love you, Mum."

16. "Thanks for being here, Mum. I love you."

17. Jy said, "I declare you the best mummy ever" and gave me a star sticker.

18. "You are the bestest mummy."

19. "I love you to infinity, Mum."

20. "I'll teach you everything I know, Jodi." I smirked and had a laugh to myself.

21. I took Jy to the park, and he started talking to a four-year-old girl and she asked me if I was a mum or a nan. I said, "I am a mum." Jy said, "My Mum is forty-one and she knows lots of things."

22. I was pushing Jy on the swing at the park and he asked me to push him as high as the building. So I pushed him as fast as I could and he said, "Mum, my

heart is excited."

23. While at the park, Jy told me he had a secret to tell me and he whispered it to me and asked me not to tell anyone. I told him I would keep his secret, and he said, "Thanks Mum." It's in the vault, my boy.

24. Jy asked me if I could buy him the Smurfs movie on DVD and I said, "No, because I don't have enough money with me." Jy said, "I have an idea, Mum," and proceeded to the kitchen drawer and collected a few dollars' worth of coins. He came back to me counting the money and asked how many coins we needed to buy the movie.

25. Jy asked me if he could have some chocolate M&Ms and I said, "Yes," and I got them for him out of the fridge. When I gave them to him, he ate them and said, "That didn't even fill my toes, Mum." Jy generally describes how full he is from his toes up to his neck.

26. Jy and I were playing pretend supermarkets in the garage with a toy counter and cash register. Jy said he wanted to be the shop person first. I said hello and asked if he could help me. I said, "Would you be able to suggest any ideas for what I can buy my five-year-old son? He said, "Hmm," and tapped his forefinger on

his cheek. "Nine chocolate eggs." Jy loves his chocolate eggs. We then swapped roles, and I was the assistant and I asked what he wanted to buy and he said as he looked around, "A trailer, a bike, a car." I asked how much money he had and he said $33."

27. I bought Jy some slime, and he loved playing with it. He put slime over his toy dinosaur's head and it was dripping down. Jy said, "Mum, take a photo and send it to all your friends." I have a real boy on my hands.

28. "You are the prettiest mummy I've ever had in a thousand years."

29. Jy woke and the first thing he said to me was, "You are my favourite mummy."

30. "How many more times do I have to go to school, Mummy?" I responded thirteen years and Jy started counting on his fingers until thirteen and said, "That's not so long." I explained he would be at school until he was eighteen and he said, "Will I be grown up then?" I said, "Yes." I encouraged Jy to do his best at school every time he goes there as there are lots of great things to learn.

31. I often talked to Jy about when I was five-years-old and I watch his face when he relates to what he does at this age. I told Jy about a boy when I was in kindergarten and he tripped me over. Jy asked if I could take him to that boy so he could tell him it wasn't nice to do that to his mum.

32. I picked Jy up from school and mentioned I was hot, so Jy started to blow air on me and his friend walked past. Jy said, "I'm cooling my mum down."

33. Jy and I were grocery shopping and Jy noticed a young boy was alone and crying. Jy asked if we could take the child home as he had no family. I said while that is a kind thought and I was proud of him for being a caring boy, we should find his parents. Which we did.

34. Jy was in the lounge room as I was making the bed in the bedroom. I walked back in the lounge room to find that Jy had got his craft scissors and cut strings on the blinds. I caught Jy in the act and asked him to please not cut the blinds and he said, "But Mum, I don't want a blind on that window anymore."

35. When Jy was four, he said he would buy me something sparkly, and I asked if it was a pair of earrings or a necklace and he said, "No, I want to buy

you a sparkly dress." I thanked him for his kindness. He said he wanted me to wear it when I marry him. I said boys don't marry their mummies, but they will always be by their son's side. I said some people get married when they are grown ups and others don't. I explained that to marry someone you must have a mutual respect of love and trust and treat them like no other as they are the one who chose their life to be with you. I said if they get married, it is to someone they have met when they grow up. He said, "Uh okay, Mum. Sorry I can't marry you."

36. Jy was displaying behaviour that needed to be addressed. I said I still love you but I would like you to make better choices and he said, "Thanks Mum, I will make better choices. Thanks for still loving me."

37. I had a routine blood test and Jy supported me by saying, "Mum, just be brave!"

38. Jy woke one morning at 4.30am and asked me if his heart stopped beating and I answered it hadn't. Jy asked for my hand and put it on his heart and I left it there and he fell back to sleep and his sweetness and innocence amazed me.

39. Jy advised me he wished he had a rocket so he

could go to Jupiter and back to planet Earth.

40. I was driving Jy to swimming lessons and there was a rainbow in the sky in front of us. It was perfectly positioned. If we kept driving, it would have felt like we would have driven straight under it. I said to Jy that I love the rainbow and he said, "Where, Mum?" I said, "Right in front of us." Jy said, "I love you more than that rainbow," and smiled at me when he saw my happy face.

41. Jy was having a shower and drew a picture of him and me on the shower screen. He drew an upside U, with another upside down U on top, with a circle on top of that. He did this twice, side by side each other. Next he drew four arms next to the middle section and two that held hands. Then he drew a love heart in between the two circle heads and said, "That's us, Mum!" I said I loved his drawing and it makes me happy because we are holding hands and love each other. He was so connected to my praise his eyes opened wide, and he had a proud look on his face.

42. I burned my lip checking Jy's milk temperature. He got a towel and patted my mouth and stopped once he was satisfied he'd cooled my lip.

43. As I was taking Jy to school and waiting for the bell to go, he was playing with his school friend, fell over and grazed his arm. I took him to the front office, and they placed a band-aid over the graze. As I walked Jy back to the assembly area, he said he can't lift anything heavy now. Could I walk him to class and could I tell the man (my manager) I was late because Jy hurt his arm.

44. Jy asked me if I would like to dance when we were in the lounge room and I said, "Okay." He said, "No, you have to say 'certainly.'" So I said, "Certainly," and we danced.

45. After collecting Jy from school one day he played tag with one of his friends and they asked me to play. So, I started chasing them around the playground and I was chasing Jy's friend. Jy yelled out really loud, "Get him, Mum! Well done, Mum!" Then he told his friends I was so good at playing tag.

46. When we went shopping, Jy wanted to look at toys. Jy knew we couldn't buy every time we went out, so this trip we were just looking. Jy found a toy, picked it up and scanned it, and it was $39. He looked at me and said, "We don't have that much money, do we, Mum?" Before I could answer, he kissed the toy, put it

back and said, "Seems like I can't buy you today."

47. When Jy was five years and three months old, I picked him up from school and he randomly asked me where he was born. I asked him if he would like me to take him to the hospital where he was born and he said yes. So, we spontaneously drove to the Hospital in Canberra. We walked through the reception area and I asked if it would be okay to show my son around as he'd just asked me if I could show him where he was born. The staff were so lovely and agreed. I walked as close as I could to the theatre and explained behind those doors I was so happy when Jy was born I cried. He said, "You cried happy tears, Mummy," and I said, "Yes, I sure did Jy." I then took Jy to the nursery and we watched from outside the window. I explained babies who need special monitoring attend the nursery, and he was a special baby. I walked him up the corridor heading towards the room I stayed in following Jy's birth. The nurse had a stethoscope and Jy asked if he could listen to her heart and they ended up listening to each other's hearts. The room I stayed in was occupied, so I sat down outside and explained to Jy behind that door is where he spent his first few days of his life. I was so touched by Jy's maturity and interest in where he was born. I don't know where his request came from, but it didn't matter. It was a beautiful afternoon

spent with a little boy five years on.

48. I was driving Jy to school, and he said whoever doesn't speak on the way to school is the winner. We both kept silent, and I pretended to zip my mouth shut and tried to talk. When we got to school Jy said, "I heard you tried to talk through your closed mouth, Mum, so that makes me the winner. But I don't want you to be the loser, so we can both be winners, I don't mind."

49. Jy was due for a haircut and the previous time had lightning bolts cut into his hair and said it made him go really fast like Buzz Lightyear from the movie Toy Story. I mentioned to Jy I would get some chocolate frogs and take him for a haircut. Jy said, "Chocolate frogs are my favourite, but mums are better and that's you. Can you get your hair cut with lightning bolts so you can be like me?"

50. Jy noticed I was typing on my laptop and he asked what I was doing. I said, "I'm typing a book about you." Jy asked, "Can I type some please, Mum?" I said, "Of course, you can." So, here is my son, Jy. Abcdefghijklmnopqrstuvwxyz. 1234567891011121314 15161718192021222324252627282930313233343536 37383940414243444546474849505152535455565758 59

606162636465666768697071727374757677787980818
28384858687888990919293949596979899100.

51. Jy got the calendar down from the wall and started crossing off the days and chose a date three weeks ahead and asked if that could be his birthday. He said it wasn't so far away and he couldn't just keep having sleeps and no birthday. His friends were having their six-year-old birthday parties, but Jy would have to wait another six months. I decided when Jy turned exactly five years and six months old we would have a small cake and sing happy five and a half years to him. This helped break the long year and the countdown he was having to endure to reach six. Why not break the rules, hey? After all, Jy and I were used to pushing the boundaries together.

52. We went camping with my family and friends. We taught Jy how to ride his bike without training wheels. He was getting a little frustrated, but he persevered and was so proud of himself when he mastered it. He kept practising and riding up the dirt road singing songs to himself. On the same trip, my family showed Jy how to cook damper in the ground and all the tricks of camping. We camped on a river bank and I took Jy up the river in the canoe. I sat in the back and rowed us along. Jy was looking up to the trees on the side of the

river bank and said, "Mum, I've never done this before and this is the best day of my life." This made me feel happy and proud that Jy was out in nature and feeling so happy.

53. On this same canoe ride, Jy noticed lots of trees and I said we need trees as they produce oxygen and we need this for energy. Jy said, "I haven't had any 'breathes' so I should have some," and started taking deep breaths through his nose.

54. On the way home from this camping holiday, Jy asked me if he could put the window down in the car as he wanted to be like Scooby Doo. Jy watched Scooby Doo the night before and Scooby was sitting in the car with his tongue flapping out the window in the wind. Yes, Jy did just that!

55. After I picked Jy up from school, I said to him the first person to see a red car (having already seen one), gets a chocolate frog when we get home. I let Jy see the red car before I did. He was so proud of himself. We played the game with different coloured cars and I let Jy spot them first. Jy then asked if he could choose the colour car and I said, "Yes for sure." So, Jy said, "Whoever spots the white car gets a hundred chocolate frogs." I knew I was about to lose this game because Jy

then said, "White car," quickly followed by, "I spotted it first, Mum" and smirked at me.

56. I was putting Jy to bed one night, and he asked me where my dad was. I felt an instant lump in the back of my throat. I explained my dad had a sick heart and passed away when I was thirty-four. I told him my dad was a wonderful man, and he loved me very much. Although Jy wasn't born when he died, he would have loved him the same way he loved me. I said he used to look after me and put me to bed like I was doing with Jy. He asked me what he used to say to me and I said he would read books to me. Jy then changed the tone of his voice to a lower tone pretending to be my dad and read the 'Three Little Pigs' story book to me. He asked what else Dad would say to me at bedtime and I said that he was proud of me and he loved me. Jy lowered his voice again and said, "I'm proud of you Jodi and I love you." Jy asked again what else happened. I said, "Dad would hold my hand and kiss me on the forehead and say goodnight." Jy again pretended to be Dad, held my hand, kissed my forehead and said, "I love you my girl." It was in the dark and I didn't let Jy see my tears, but I was overwhelmed at what my boy was saying. I wanted my dad to be near me again and Jy's interest that night about him made me feel Dad was close to me again.

57. Jy discovered my phone had a recording function. So, he sang songs to me and recorded them. "Let's name this one, 'Mum is so pretty'. 'Mum is so pretty and I love her much.'" (Repeated.)

58. Jy was playing on his computer and I held his hand and then tried to let go. Jy wanted me to hold his hand as he played his computer. Of course, I stopped typing this book and held his hand.

59. An ad came on TV about skydiving. I skydived when I was thirty and was explaining this to Jy as I often talked to him about things I've done in my life. Jy asked if I did this when he was in my tummy and I said no and that would be too dangerous to do if he was in my tummy. He asked if my brain was still deciding to have him and I said, "Yes."

60. Jy wanted me to get something he left in the car only two minutes after I woke one morning. I said I will in a second, I just need to wake up properly. Within seconds, Jy said, "Mum, it's been one second," and I said he was correct and could he just give me five minutes and I explained one second was a figure of speech. He said, "Why didn't you tell me that when I was four because I thought I knew everything already."

61. Jy said, "Mum, if anyone says you are 1000 great, I'll tell them that you are one million great."

62. When Jy was five, he wanted to help me more at home. I filmed Jy helping me and he said, "Merry Christmas Santa, I'm going to make a surprise for you. I'm helping Mumma to pack up the house, Santa because I'm growing up. The end. Santa is going to like it!" Yes, it was around Christmas time and Jy wanted to help me but also impress the fella in the red suit.

63. I had a sore back so Jy offered to help me carry some bags and massaged my back. He said he will make me better and handed me the phone so I could call Santa to let him know Jy had been good.

64. Jy did something he didn't think was nice to me so he said, "I am saying sorry eight times because I wasn't fair to you."

65. Jy and I were sitting in a stationary ute and I said I really liked this car. Jy said, "I do too, Mum, but where will my wife and children sit?"

66. Jy was playing I Spy with me. He was sitting on the toilet at the time and said, "BK." I had to guess was it was and couldn't. Jy asked, "Give up, Mum?" I said

yes and Jy said, "It was butt crack, Mum."

67. I took Jy to the local carnival and after he went on the oversized dragon slide, he said, "This is the best day of my life".

68. Jy, Mum, Aunty Kathy and I were in my car. It was a gas car that had made a noise when it started and you could a see puff of gas come out from under the bonnet. Jy was in the back seat and heard the noise and said, "Moke, Mummy, Moke!" Jy thought the gas cloud was fire and was trying to say there was smoke!

69. I was about to say to Jy 'I love you,' and he said, "I love you as much as you love me."

70. Jy told me he was digging for diamonds in the playground at school so he could make me a ring.

71. Jy and I were having a movie night at home and the rocket was about to blast off in the movie. Jy held me and said, "Mum, I'll give you a cuddle because the rocket noise will scare you!"

72. I bought Jy a new toy and he said, "Thank you Mummy, you are my dynamite girl."

73. Jy said he will be a billionaire when he is older and can buy a Ferrari so he can drive to me faster if I'm having a heart attack like my dad did.

74. Jy said if one of us goes to heaven, our love won't break because our hearts are connected and he gave me a cuddle so our chests touched.

75. At Jy's sixth birthday party, he said I was the best mum that has ever walked on planet Earth.

76. Mum inducted her grandchildren into what she called, 'Nanna's Elvis Hall of Fame.' During car rides to school, I would play Elvis' 'Viva Las Vegas.' I taught Jy the words and called Mum one day to let her listen to Jy sing the song. Jy was really getting into it. It was funny, and I recorded it to add to his collection of his magic moments.

77. I was delighted to be served breakfast in bed by Jy. He gave me one piece of toast with a bite taken out of it.

78. I was feeling unwell and I noticed Jy went to the kitchen and got me a cup of water. He wrote 'I love you Mum' on a piece of paper and stuck it to the cup. He put a straw into the cup and brought it to me and said,

"This will make you feel better Mummy."

79. Jy advised me one morning upon waking that he was going to be the Prime Minister when he is older. He said he will create ideas that don't cause pollution and give all children free toys.

80. Following school, Jy gave me a ring made from his broken shoelace. He gave it to me and said, "I love you more, Mum."

81. Jy was reading the chapter list for this book. After he finished, I proudly declared that if I didn't have him in my life, I wouldn't have been able to write this book and reminded him how incredibly precious he was. He said, "Thank you Mum. You really love me, Mum, but I love you more."

82. When I was settling Jy into bed, he asked me what date my Dad passed away and I said 4th July 2008. Jy then said he will make a time machine to go back to the day before my Dad died to take him to hospital so the doctors can stop his heart attack.

83. My mum returned from a doctor's visit to find out a lump the doctor removed from her neck was a skin cancer. Jy said to Mum, "Are you OK, Nan? Please

keep checking for skin cancers because I want you to be OK."

84. Jy told me that his gut feeling predicts the future and in three seconds he will say "I love you." Then he said, "I love you, Mum. See! My gut feeling was right."

85. When Jy was 3.5 years old, I took him to a festival and he sat in the front of a fire truck. The next day, he decided he was going to save the world. He wanted to be Fireman Sam and advised me I was Fire Lady Sam. He placed a bungee cord around his waist as a fireman's belt and had a spirit level as his ladder. Jy asked me to drive the fire truck (cubby house steering wheel) and to slow at the orange light, stop at the red light and turn right when the light goes green. Then he asked me to get out and rescue the girl crying for her mummy. He then told me that I did a good job and put his thumb up in appreciation. I heard him answer the cubby house phone and said, "What's happening? This road is really bumpy. We are on our way, weeeeeooooooor, weeeeooooorrrr!" Then he locked me in the cubby house and said, "C'mon team, we need to rescue my Mum!"

86. While driving to school, Jy put his arm forward with a closed fist and said, "My mum has superpowers!"

87. Who needs a warm bed when you have a warm mum?

88. When Jy was very young and was going to bed, he said, "Blankey on, Mummy," which meant he wanted me to tuck him into bed.

89. Jy asked me if he could not go to school today as he wanted to take me to the moon.

90. I was dealing with a difficult situation I'd shielded Jy from for many years. Through no fault of Jy's or mine, the future I'd planned and envisaged for us both was derailed. As a result, my strength and determination to create a great life for Jy and me, the same determination I used to get Jy, led us to a magical place—a place we both deserved to be.

I never showed anything but strength and love to Jy. This particular night I was shedding a tear because I felt Jy deserved better and I didn't realise Jy noticed. He sat beside me, patted my back and said, "Mum, take a deep breath and calm down." Then he wiped my tears with the sleeve of his shirt and gave me a cuddle and kiss. I was so impressed with his compassion at such a young age. I'd invested so much in Jy to develop his emotional wellbeing, and this beautiful child before me was showing compassion beyond his years. I praised Jy for being so kind and making me feel better.

I told Jy that sometimes tears are happy tears, and Mummy was feeling extremely happy. In fact, I couldn't wipe the smile off my face. I was also so proud at what I'd fought for. When a door closes (which I'd slammed shut), I believe in opening a window. Even if it's difficult to open, you go by belief and not sight. I displayed sheer determination, strength, living in my powerful truth, exuding confidence and self-belief. I was proudly and happily driving my life.

I kicked goal after goal and placed our future back on track for both of us. Our future together would forever shine and it became so bright we had to wear shades!

Photos of Jy

Two embryos implanted. Jy is one of them

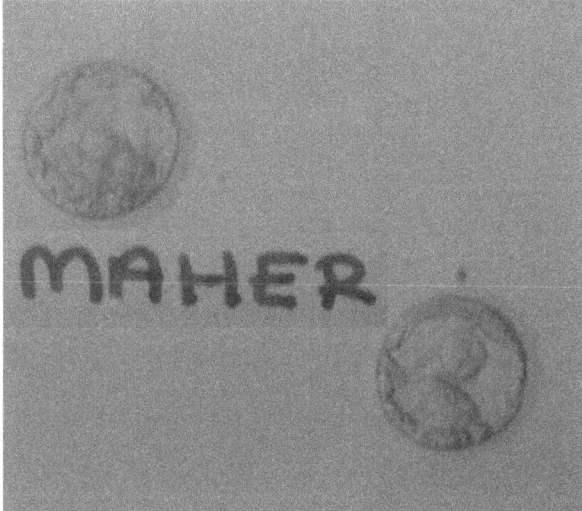

Jy displaying the peace sign during an ultrasound

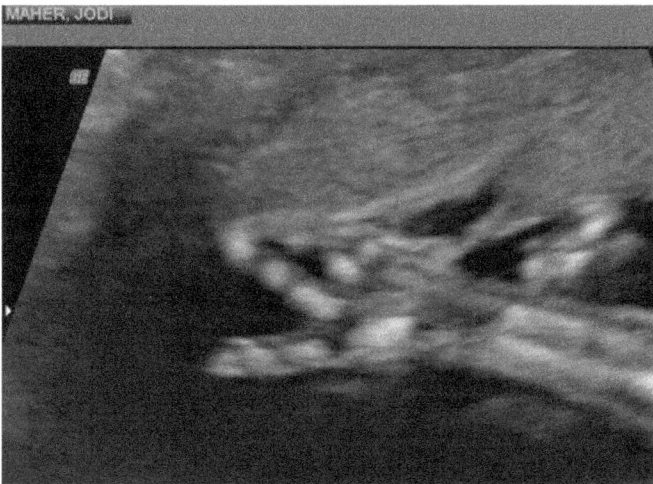

Holding Jy for the first time. He has one eye open

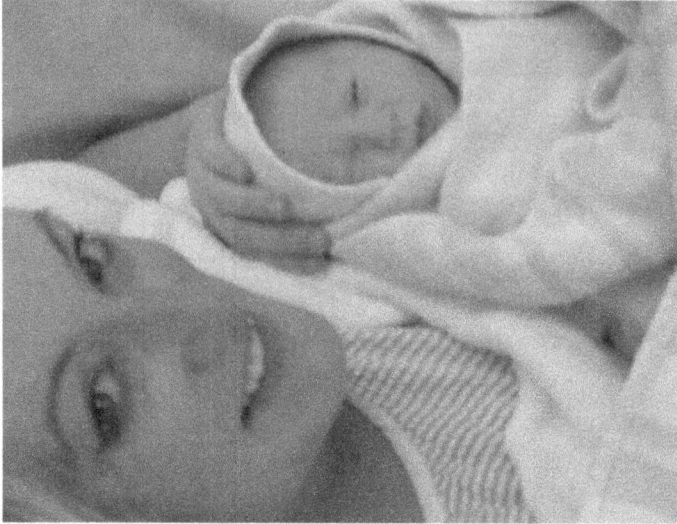

Jy two days old in the hospital bassinette

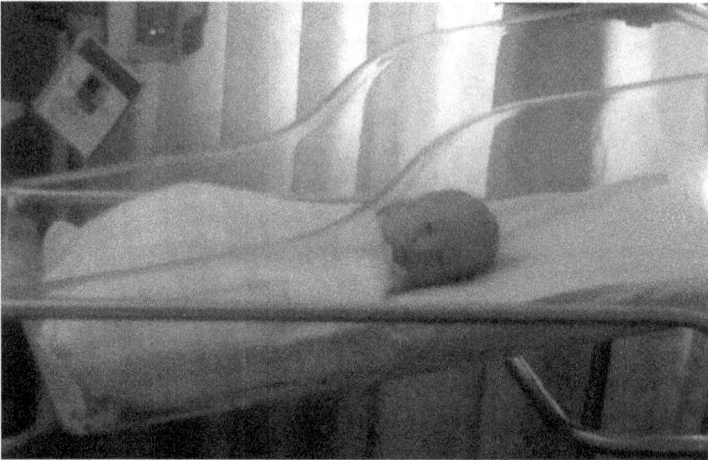

Taking Jy home from hospital following his birth

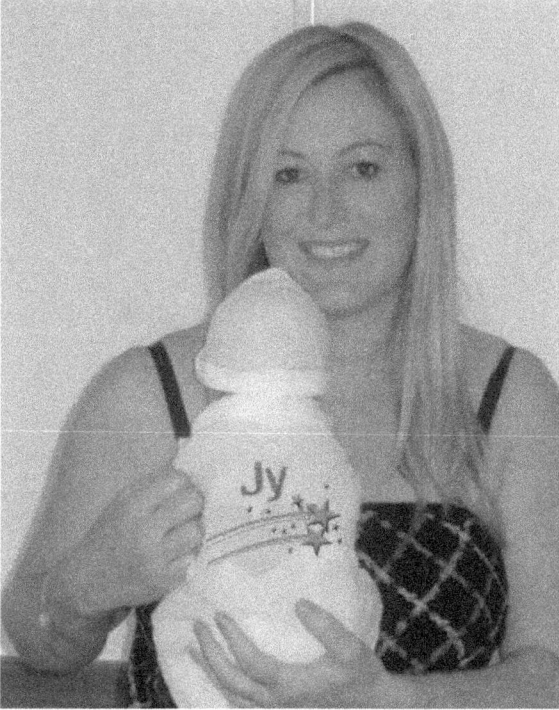

4D pregnancy scan of Jy and the same profile when he was a few months old

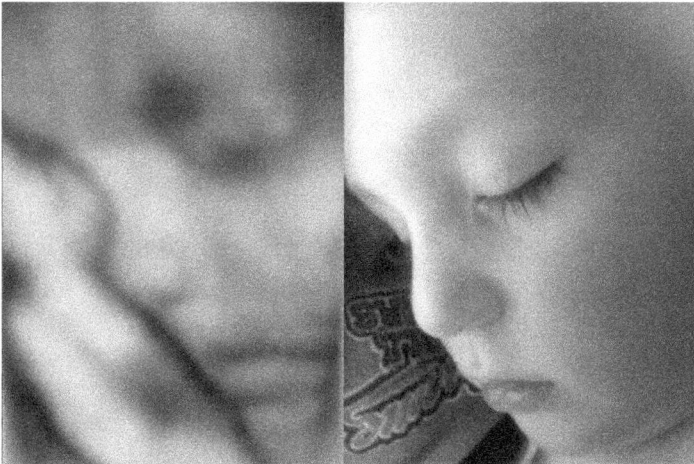

Nursing Jy through his 12 month sickness

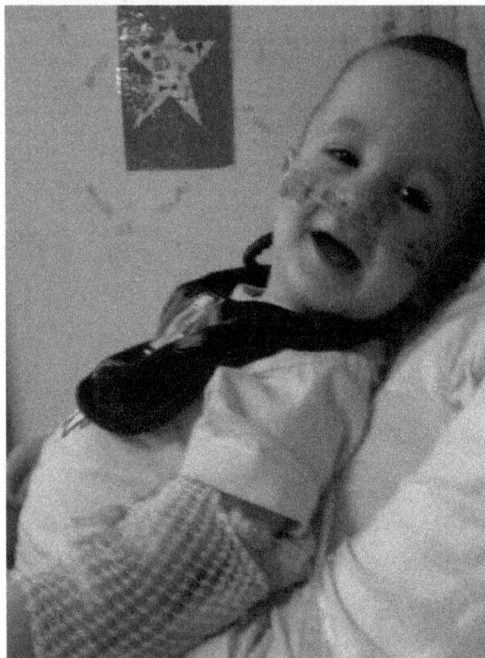

Jy's first day of pre school

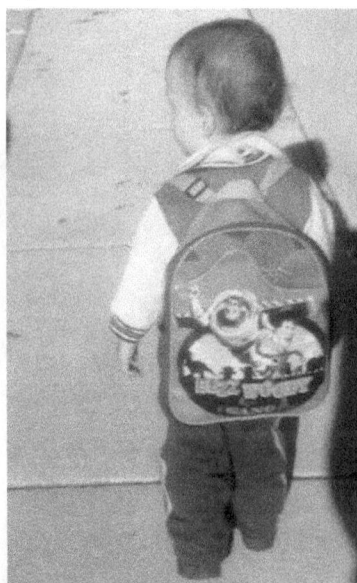

CHAPTER TWENTY-SIX

A light that forever shines

As part of establishing a brand new, bright and exciting life, Jy started at a new school. He was feeling quite nervous to do so. I thought he was so brave and knew he would love the activities on offer. I gave Jy a massive hug and encouraged him to have a great first day at his new school. I went to work and when I returned to collect Jy at the end of the school day, his little face lit up. He said, "Mummy, I have a new friend named Zachary and I like my teacher." That made me feel so happy that my little one appeared to be settled.

Zachary was a boy who seemed to light up the world around him. He'd a calm and friendly manner, and Jy told me he couldn't wait to go to school the next day to see Zachary.

After some time, I met Zachary's Mum. Kim contacted me as Jy had given Zachary his computer game to borrow for the night. Kim tracked me down to let me know she will take care of the device and return it with Zachary tomorrow.

I explained to Kim how supportive and kind Zachary was to Jy and expressed my gratitude. Zachary's kindness helped me as an adult to know my precious little boy had met someone kind at school who would look out for him.

I could see where Zachary got his kindness. Kim just radiated beauty and warmth and was always supporting Jy and I. At this point, I did not know how brightly Zachary shone his light and changed the entire direction of his mum's life.

I later mentioned to Kim that Jy was born following 11 rounds of IVF and she was mesmerised and could not believe I'd attempted so many rounds to have one child. You never can tell the heartache a person has been through by looking at them. People did not know my deep sadness as I went through painstaking and heartbreaking moments with IVF.

I was completely shocked about what Kim would tell

me next. Kim shared with me that she had six precious little cherubs in Heaven and four babies on Earth, and this stopped me in my tracks. Kim reminded me of the lady whose story moved me throughout IVF, with a common number of babies being ten.

From a young age, Kim knew she wanted a big family. She adored children but was sad to be advised by a medical professional at sixteen that she wouldn't be able to fall pregnant due to PCOS that caused malignant cysts. Doctors made Kim aware at this point that she might require a full hysterectomy at a younger age. This was overwhelming and extremely difficult for Kim to process.

For some time, Kim tried to adapt to the medical opinion, but this gave her more determination to fulfil her deep primal desire to become a mother. Kim wanted a big family.

With a loving husband Damien and some years later, Kim proved this medical opinion wrong.

When Kim found out she was pregnant for the first time, she was in a state of happiness, shock and absolutely delighted that they were going to become parents. However, the fear was overwhelming because

Kim was told explicitly that it was not going to happen. Living with this fear and wondering if Kim's body would hold the pregnancy was consuming.

This elation soon turned to sadness when Kim had signs of a miscarriage. She rushed to her doctor, who conducted an ultrasound where a faint heartbeat was discovered. Kim was sent home to rest, but sadly two days later, she miscarried at 11.5 weeks. This left Kim and Damien feeling devastated. Their hopes of becoming parents were dashed in an instant. While Kim felt devastated, she'd discovered she could fall pregnant. However, carrying a baby to term was where Kim's fear and anxiety really set in.

Kim felt helpless and did not know where to turn next. After trying to come to terms with this unexpected experience, Kim successfully became pregnant again. However, this little one would result in the same outcome and Kim miscarried at seven weeks. Kim was feeling the lowest of lows and wondering why this was happening to her.

Kim was left feeling winded from her loss but knew she had to carry on. With Damien by her side, they sought medical intervention and investigating other specialist opinions to give themselves the best chance to have the family they so dearly wanted.

Kim and Damien hoped for a healthy baby and at this point, they were hoping to carry a baby to term and hold their little one in their arms. They kept wishing and yearning about a little boy who might become a big brother, and the name they'd agreed on for over a decade was Zachary.

Kim was surprised and was ecstatic to discover she was pregnant again, but continued to tread carefully because she was so afraid she may miscarriage this little one too. Kim hoped and prayed this baby, who was due on her wedding anniversary, would grow beautifully and make it to full term.

This pregnancy advanced without complication, and following an ultrasound that confirmed a heartbeat, Kim and Damien were thrilled to notify close friends for the first time that they would be having a baby.

At fourteen weeks, Kim was shattered when her body gave her no warning that this little baby had passed. Despite knowing the doctors informed Kim she couldn't fall pregnant, the pattern of losing three little babies was clear. It was Kim's new reality. Maybe the doctors were right.

At this moment, with Damien's constant support, Kim's dismay was she secretly worried she would never become a mother. Kim felt she was robbing Damien of a chance to become a father, and this drove Kim to keep investigating medical options to create their family.

Coming to terms with this reality hit Kim incredibly hard, and it took some time for Kim to come to terms that this little one couldn't stay. Kim felt alone and worried if she would ever become a mother. What would a future look like with no children when all you want is children? This reality was the reason Kim felt she needed to give this baby an identity as she feared she may continue to have babies who she wasn't lucky enough to ever meet. This little heartbeat was named Henry. Kim quietly kept the name Zachary reserved in her heart, in the event that one day, she may actually hold him.

Kim realised she may need to consider alternate options, including adoption and fostering children as a mum is a mum to any baby/child in Kim's eyes.

While processing these options, Kim knew the only way forward would be to keep trying to create her family. Her celebration was stunted with incredible worry when she became pregnant for a fourth time.

She was afraid and felt the miscarriages were affecting her ability to feel at peace. Kim tried to carry on as normal, giving each pregnancy a brand new chance to develop into a beautiful healthy baby. She ate well and took care of herself to ensure she was giving this baby every chance of success.

Kim passed the gestation of her longest pregnancy to date and started to believe that she may carry this baby full term. She unravelled some happy feelings, however she kept reserved because of her fear of losing another baby. Kim's regular scans revealed her wishes were granted. She had a healthy baby on board and was fast approaching her second trimester. Kim sat and reflected about her little babies she'd lost. She felt she owed it to them to keep trying. She wanted to honour their lives lost by trying to keep going and being emotionally strong and focussed.

Kim was feeling content and dreaming about meeting her baby. Her fourth baby was on board and within weeks, Kim would become a mother. It had been a long and painful process to get to this joyful moment, and she was so proud of what Damien and she achieved.

Kim had a standard medical appointment at thirty-seven weeks to check her baby and was advised to go home and pack her bags as she would have a baby tomorrow. Kim required medical assistance to induce the birth. She was so frightened because she needed her body to hang on a little longer as Kim felt solely responsible for this baby arriving safely into the world.

Kim's thoughts turned to yearning for the cry. The baby's cry that women need to hear. That first cry that says their baby has arrived. Kim felt so afraid her body would let her down, but felt so close. She trusted her obstetrician that if he had to deliver her baby safely, by any means, he would save both their lives.

Kim's midwife had previously explained the birthing process to Kim, answering Kim's question of how will she know when the baby was on its way. Her midwife reassured her that she would know and that moment had just arrived.

Kim was ready to push and knew she would meet her baby within minutes. Time then stood still. Kim and Damien held their breath in anticipation and waited for the sound they'd been hoping to hear for years. Their baby boy sucked in all his air and let out the biggest cry and Kim broke down in tears because she realised her baby had made it and was safe.

Zachary was handed to his mum for the first time, while his Dad cut the cord. Kim's fourth baby had left her bursting with happiness and tears were rolling down her face and she quietly reflected that as a family, they'd made it! Kim and Damien felt so relieved and incredibly grateful for this precious child that instantly beamed light in their world.

Zachary was handed to Damien, and it was discovered soon after that the obstetrician had also delivered Damien when he was born, which brought absolute delight to deliver two generations in one family.

Kim and Damien found success with Zachary, which gave them the confidence they needed to try again, despite the initial medical diagnosis. Kim discovered she was pregnant for the fifth time. Her chances were 25% odds of a successful pregnancy based on one live birth from four pregnancies. Kim knew that this could go either way, and this time the odds weren't favourable. Sadly, Kim lost this little one at ten weeks. Another baby was gone.

A little while later, Kim had some medical issues and was admitted to hospital for surgery which involved inserting a stent. Damien, as always, was a magnificent support and was caring for Zachary while Kim was sick in hospital. This helped Kim to relax as best as she could, knowing her bright light was in good hands with his dad.

As the doctors were examining Kim post-operation, they conducted an ultrasound and discovered Kim was pregnant, which was delightful news but immediately was considered a troubling scenario. This worried Kim and her doctor because of Kim's health predicament.

Kim felt incredibly blessed to be pregnant again, but was nervous and worried about her own health and that of her baby. With pregnancy number six growing while Kim was on bedrest, both Kim and her doctors were quite concerned when Kim showed signs of miscarriage.

Sadly, an ultrasound confirmed Kim had lost this baby too. Kim sat in her hospital bed reflecting on how each one of her precious babies had a heartbeat. To date, Kim had six babies, with one she could hold in her arms.

Zachary forever shone his bright light since the day he was born and constantly reminded his parents of how incredibly precious one heart beat reaching full term was.

It would soon become a reality that Zachary would fulfil the big brother role Damien and Kim often envisaged.

CHAPTER TWENTY-SEVEN
Ten Heartbeats

A few weeks later, during post-surgery check-up and preparation for the removal of the stent, it was discovered by blood test and ultrasound that Kim was nine weeks pregnant. This was confusing and shocked Kim because previously she sensed she may be pregnant, but this time was there was no indication. The heartbeat was the gestation of the sixth baby she'd lost, which meant Kim had been pregnant with twins and had lost one. This realisation was overwhelming for Kim, yet astounding to know how brilliant the human body is, including this resilient and stubborn little soul who remained onboard as Kim's seventh heartbeat, while she recovered from surgery.

This pregnancy would prove difficult as the growth measurements were of concern. Kim was incredibly sick and while in hospital, she asked for a tracing machine to let her know her baby was still with her. They also discovered the scar tissue on Kim's uterus wouldn't allow the uterus to expand, causing the secondary issue of amniotic fluid leaking. This can lead to the risk of a dry birth, increasing the chances of her baby dying in utero, which may explain earlier miscarriages. To avoid this risk, they gave Kim the option and she agreed to get a stitch at twenty-four weeks to give this pregnancy the best chance of survival.

After what felt like forever, this little baby kept hanging on and as a result, it inspired Kim to do everything within her means to feel positive and have hope. This baby lived through a twin dying, two of Kim's surgeries, and was defying Kim's track record of lack of success with pregnancies. For the first time, Kim felt like this little baby would be a girl. With such a fierce and strong will to survive, Kim felt she must be having a daughter.

Kim was at the hospital for a check-up and was advised because of low amniotic fluid, this baby would need to be induced tomorrow. This was the same scenario Kim found herself in with Zachary. Kim felt she was slightly more prepared this time around and it was reassuring that Kim had to, again, believe in herself.

The following day, at 36.6 weeks, a baby girl named Scarlett safely entered the world. Kim and Damien felt so blessed to have two healthy children.

Scarlett was an unsettled baby with projectile reflux and requiring two hourly feeds, which she gulped down. The doctors medicated her at four weeks of age and placed her on solid food early at four months as her body didn't appear to be accepting the nutrition. As the weeks went on, Scarlett would continue to have episodes where she would become pale and floppy after her feeds, and these severe reactions only continued to get worse. She was feeding differently to Zachary, and Kim suspected something was very wrong. Kim immediately obtained an appointment with a new paediatrician who conducted several tests.

One day, Scarlett became so unwell, they admitted her to hospital. After being examined, medical staff were concerned she was not on the chart for her height and weight and as a result, they took Kim aside and questioned her about neglecting her baby because of her size. Scarlett was wearing four zero baby clothes at eight months old. Kim understood the line of questioning and appreciated the vigilance of medical staff to protect children. Because of Scarlet's size, Kim urged the doctors to dig deeper as she knew her daughter had much more than reflux.

After weeks of tests and procedures, they diagnosed Scarlett with two conditions. Eosinophilic esophagitis known as EOE, which is a chronic allergic/immune condition of the oesophagus, and Food Protein Induced Enterocolitis Syndrome known as FPIES. These conditions caused a collection of cells to form little tumours at the base of Scarlett's oesophagus. They'd turned malignant. Scarlett would require immediate surgery and was appointed an oncologist by her immunologist (who still calls Scarlett 'Poppet' to this day). Scarlett's surgery saw doctors remove an incredible 17milimetres of her oesophagus.

Check-ups and surgeries became the new normal for this courageous little girl. For the next two years, Scarlett lived solely on a liquid only diet, a unique formula that gave her the nutrients she needed to grow whilst being safe for her body. Scarlett gets scared and uptight when she approaches hospitals because of the numerous treatments she has undertaken in her young years.

Scarlett has been part of many medical food trials and diets. When Scarlett was diagnosed, she was one of the first cases in Australia for her treating immunologist. There are now hundreds. Scarlett's story and agreement to participate in medical studies is to inform doctors, but also is in the hope to extend her life expectancy and others.

Scarlett is like a little mother and dotes over babies. This is something Kim hopes can become a reality in Scarlett's life one day if she can overcome the odds and technology advances. If her spirit and strength are anything to go by, she will certainly beat the odds.

With two beautiful children, Kim and Damien decided to try again to increase their family as they had so much love to give and both felt they wanted more children. Kim had blissfully fallen pregnant with her eighth baby, and all tests and scans were marking milestones.

As with all Kim's losses, what happened next hit her hard and this heartbeat in particular, left a gaping hole in her heart. Sadly, a beautiful baby which Kim named Willow was born at nineteen weeks gestation. Kim remembers a beautiful butterfly on the door of the delivery suite. This became Kim's eight heartbeat and sixth angel.

A few weeks later, they celebrated Scarlett's first

birthday and were so grateful their little girl, despite the rough start, was finding her way in the world. Scarlett continued to be strong and fight with all her might, responding with such resilience after each procedure. Kim and Damien also decided they would try for one more baby and this would be their last attempt.

To their absolute delight, they found out Kim was pregnant with their ninth heartbeat. The worry of which way this pregnancy would go would being a constant thought process for them to manage. Kim knew how vulnerable this world of pregnancy was and needed to take it a day at a time and be prepared for any outcome.

Kim was feeling trepidation because of the same complications as she progressed in weeks with Zachary and Scarlett's pregnancies, being low fluid, and her uterus not growing.

At the same time, Kim felt calmer in the sense of nerves, fears and insecurities. She was petrified knowing that not only miscarriage, which is so painful to deal with, but also her baby born sleeping had been added to Kim's list of fears. Kim tuned into her intuition and reminded herself to be realistic as nothing is certain. She talked to her heartbeat and said she would do everything within her power to protect this little one. Kim couldn't bring herself to feel at ease or confident until she heard this heartbeat cry. She was trying to protect her own heart from a pain she knew would break her for the last time, should she have lost her ninth heartbeat.

Kim and Damien's third live birth resulted in the delivery room being fill with joy. A baby boy named Lachlan entered the world so fast, the midwives all nicknamed him Cannonball.

Lachlan birthed so fast; his body couldn't regulate the level of oxygen. They whisked him away to the special care nursery when he remained for a few days. Kim recalls screaming at Damien from the bed where she delivered Lachlan, with angst and worry, to remind him to stay by Lachlan's side.

Because of the scar tissue within Kim's uterus, it couldn't contract, which generally stops the excess bleeding once the placenta is birthed. Kim's uterus had essentially broken. It failed to do as it should have, and her body haemorrhaged. It became quite a blur for Kim as she needed to have a blood transfusion.

Over the following weeks, Lachlan was what Kim

always called her colour-changing skittle. He would go from yellow to orange to pink to purple, all in the space of a day. It took him some weeks to settle down and for his body to regulate itself independently. After a full clearance of health, Lachlan left hospital, which was the most magical feeling for Kim and Damien. He'd made Kim and Damien feel they'd achieved the family they envisaged in their hearts and set out to create.

The time spent after Lachlan was born made Kim feel nostalgic. Kim's Poppy often called her his Macleay baby, after where he lived near the Macleay River when growing up. He often told Kim she was the apple of his eye and although he passed away when Kim was young, he still held such a strong presence in Kim's life and still does to this day. It only seemed fitting to honour her Poppy and include this name for their last boy's middle name.

Lachlan reminds Kim of her Pop. He is an old soul, incredibly smart and very reserved. The epitome of a quiet achiever. He loves to tinker, work things out and understand how the world around him grows. He loves a good game of chess and always takes a moment to smell the roses as he passes them by. Kim feels Lachlan holds a special piece of her Poppy's honourable and hardworking soul inside his own.

With their family now complete, Kim and Damien packed up their three beautiful children, Zachary, Scarlett and Lachlan, and they went on a local family holiday. It seemed like bliss to be away from hospitals and they timed their one week holiday to fit in between Scarlett's medical appointments.

Kim had some delightful news to share with Damien. To her astonishment, they were pregnant with their tenth heartbeat. Over the next week of holidays, they would reflect on what they'd achieved, the family they'd created and their unborn child. They were at peace and excited at the prospect of the tenth heartbeat joining their family.

It seemed like Kim's body had given out during this pregnancy as she was constantly sick. At twenty-four weeks, Kim took herself to hospital where she collapsed because of medical issues, including her kidney having shut down. Kim fiercely protected her heartbeats and desire to have a family, but the realisation had occurred. Kim must put herself first and listen to her body. In an instant, Damien was being Mum and Dad at home while Kim remained in hospital for another six weeks. Kim went home for Easter Sunday to see her family while leaving lines in and returned to the hospital soon after.

With Kim still being treated, she was so grateful for the earth children she had. However, her grief and sadness consumed her. She reflected on the heartbeats she would never get to meet and was fearing this baby on board may still share their same fate. Her tenth heartbeat would then kick, which helped ease her aching heart.

This pregnancy felt different for Kim. While as incredibly precious as all her heartbeats, this baby was a beautiful surprise. The joy of feeling her last heartbeat kicking were moments Kim relished, and watching her pregnant stomach grow for the last time was a beautiful time.

As she was so unwell, Kim became a permanent residence of the maternity ward. All eyes were constantly on Kim's baby, via monitors, traces and blood tests, to ensure the statistics were known every single minute.

Knowing Kim was living and being monitored in hospital until the day they delivered her baby brought Kim peace, and a sense of unique security and deepest gratitude. Kim was astounded she was alive, but somehow this precious little blessing was too. It was now out of her hands. Kim wished and hoped for a great outcome.

While still feeling sick, her obstetrician advised Kim at her usual daily check-up that this baby will be born today. Kim was four centimetres dilated at thirty two weeks. Her body was declining. Kim developed pre-eclampsia, the observations became irregular; the baby stopped moving and was showing reduced signs of life.

The obstetrician discussed the two delivery options and Kim was petrified about having a caesarean as she'd never had one before. Kim advised she would continue with the traditional delivery as that had been her good old faithful and they both laughed. Kim walked around the delivery suite with only the clothes on her back and called Damien.

When Kim's obstetrician put the intravenous drip in, he said, "Right, if you can make this quick, I've made a dinner reservation with my wife," and they both laughed again. It was his way to break the nervous vibe in the room.

Despite Kim's sickness, she felt so at home in the hospital ward and looked around to take in the surroundings as she knew she wouldn't be back again. The obstetrician's request was granted. One hour later, following a complication free delivery, a premature and so tiny baby boy named William was all wrapped up in Kim's arms. Kim cried many happy tears for William and felt an overwhelming sense of accomplishment that her family was complete.

Once William was born, it was like all the fear Kim ever held deep within lifted. William took fear away from his mum. He gave her the gift of complete contentment as he well and truly completed a beautiful family.

From the start, William came out running and hasn't stopped. He is laid back, calm, witty, confident, outgoing and hugs everyone he meets. Despite being the youngest, he can do exactly what his older siblings can do.

William was the baby Kim and Damien weren't expecting to have, which is a beautiful and surprising gift for families that experience loss. To not expect a baby and then have one truly is a blessing. Kim and Damien decided they weren't prepared to roll the dice again because of Kim's health concerns. They were truly blessed to have created ten heartbeats and have four beautiful children to hold.

Damien, who provided so incredibly well for his family, had supported his wife through her sickness, miscarriages, births and Scarlett's sickness. Kim described Damien as a man who never expects any credit, is absolutely incredible and she is so lucky to have such a wonderful supporting husband and father of her children.

Kim feels it's hard for society to know how to react to people's sadness associated with miscarriage and babies born sleeping. Some people are judgemental, while others do or don't know what to say. Kim knows people would have opinions, but she couldn't help that she wanted a big family. It was just what her heart desired, so she chased her desires and hopes with no guarantee or insight into how it would end up.

Kim felt the medical staff, including the same obstetrician and midwife for all deliveries over the eleven years she had her ten heartbeats, were professional, supportive, and they all changed and saved her life. Kim will forever remain a part of trials to help arm doctors with results to help them create and save lives in the future. This is her way of saying thank you for caring for her and her children.

Kim got her strength from her Poppy, her husband

and her beautiful children and until she finds her babies in heaven, they will forever be her missing pieces.

Kim's message is for women who try so incredibly hard to have a child/children is to make sure they stop and look after themselves too. As a mother or mother to be, you are so very important.

I felt numb listening to Kim's story, and we constantly remind each other to be kind to ourselves during the moments of reflection which make us cry both tears of happiness and sadness. We look at our precious babies on earth and are so grateful we can touch their little faces and hold them tight.

Kim reminds me of another beautiful woman in my life who cried many baby tears, my adorable little sister.

CHAPTER TWENTY-EIGHT
Little Sister

From the moment I punched the air when I heard Renée was born in 1984, she has brought so much love and joy to my family. I love having a younger sister.

Once Renée was ready to have children, she found herself in the same situation as me and needed to undertake IVF to have a child. Our reasons for requiring IVF were not the same, but the worry and uncertainty was.

I spoke to Mum about Renée going through IVF and she couldn't understand why both her girls needed this intervention. I explained to Mum what the medical opinion was and that it was just the way it was and if we were born generations ago, we wouldn't be able to have children. Mum said she felt as concerned but more prepared for her second daughter going through IVF. Both Mum and I became rock solid support for Renée.

I sat down with Renée and explained a whole round of IVF to her. I remember her face was amazed and I guess a little worried about what lay ahead. I told her I know she can do this.

Even though Renée knew my journey and supported me as I went through IVF, she was now experiencing the force of IVF herself. Renée got a sense of what a huge achievement it was to complete one round and hope every day for a positive result. I remember Renée's amazed face when she was coming to terms with what I went through during eleven rounds. She was in awe of what I achieved. I'd blessed her with a beautiful nephew and she was hoping to grace me with the same aunty role.

I was so proud of Renée for doing IVF because she was in an unknown world and I knew how difficult it was. I hoped with all I had my sister would not have to endure multiple rounds. I didn't want her to have to deal with the constant commitment and emotional roller coasters. I knew there was nothing more I could do except hold her up when she needed it. I was now in Mum's shoes and felt how she did when she was supporting me. I encouraged Renée to do the next step, whatever that may be, and I hoped she got a favourable result first attempt. I reassured Renée that Mum and I will be by her side every step of the way.

Once Renée was underway with the injections, she contacted me to say she didn't deposit all the liquid from the injection pen into her stomach. I think it might have been nerves. I remember my first time injecting the needle and it was nerve wrecking. After a call to the clinic, Renée felt comforted and followed their instructions.

I think the enormity of what I'd achieved was a motivating factor for Renée, who would often say she doesn't know how I did IVF eleven times. It's a mother's heart. Renée was stepping into this territory and I just couldn't wait for her to be a mother. I explained to her that maybe all my attempts were unlucky and I hoped luck would be on her side a lot sooner.

It's ironic Renée was going through IVF as I was writing parts of this book. She was asking me questions and I would send her snippets of my unfinished book and she said to me as she read it, "That's exactly how I feel."

I made the effort to contact Renée all the time, to listen to how she felt and to put her at ease. After all, I was proof IVF works. I was also mindful that for some people, IVF doesn't work. It was a fine line to walk and not get too many hopes up, while remaining a positive force.

Renée was asking me lots of questions about follicles and how many she would get each round.

She said, "Imagine if it worked first round."

I said, "I'm hoping for your sake it does, Nae."

Renée asked me if the clinic would make her wait eight weeks between rounds and I advised if that is the Specialist's policy, then yes, they would.

She said, "That would be such a long wait."

I could feel all my questions and concerns coming back through Renée now. It felt like this for me too. Eight weeks seemed like such a long time.

Renée had her last ultrasound to check on the number of follicles. I tried to prepare her in a positive way because I remembered that lady beside me during my first egg collection in round one and she didn't have any eggs in her follicles. I said to Renée the follicle numbers were good, just keep positive and what will be, will be. I was afraid to say the following to Renée, but felt I needed to be honest. I said not all the follicles will have eggs, not all eggs can be fertilised and not all embryos can survive. I explained the worst-case scenario because I knew she could handle the truth. I also explained she had a great number of follicles and let's hold on to the facts, not the 'what ifs'.

Once Renée got to egg collection day, she was relieved to have some eggs come out of the follicles. Renée got a call the same afternoon to say two eggs don't look that good. I said to Renée I was sorry, but I wasn't upset as she was still in a good position. To please look after herself and that if the embryo is strong enough, it will make it. She said okay and that it was so nerve wrecking. I knew the holding pattern she was in and I felt helpless.

I sent Renée and her husband, Adam, a message that read, "Hi Nae and Adam, just messaging you to let you know I am so proud of you both. This morning's (egg collection) is something that isn't really understood until you go through it. It's clinical. I am absolutely thrilled with your result. I hope you get pregnant and have enough to freeze for future attempts to increase your family size. Now we wait overnight to see how many cells have developed in the embryo. It's out of your hands now. Look after yourself and each other. Fantastic effort, I'm so proud of both of you. Jodi x."

Renée made it through to Day Five implant day with one Grade A embryo (the best type) and that's it. This would be her only chance this round. Fortunately, it only takes one embryo to hold a baby.

Renée was in the middle of her eleven day pregnancy result wait. She said she doesn't feel any different and asked me if she should feel anything. I advised it was normal to not feel any different and you feel as though you are getting your period even if you really weren't. Renée just wanted the outcome.

As we were all waiting with Renée and Adam during the eleven-day wait for the pregnancy result, my son was five and had fallen asleep at bedtime. I kissed his forehead and held his hand as I did the first night he was born and every night since. As I did this, I wished for Renée and Adam to be given this same chance—to kiss their child goodnight.

The days were so long and the wait seemed to take forever. Was Renée pregnant or not? I checked in daily on Renée to see how she was holding up and she said she just needed to know the result.

My phone rang on the day Renée was due to find out and I got butterflies answering the call. Little sister, you were so sweet apologising to me and being concerned for me because you had got pregnant on your first round of IVF. I could feel you were so sorry it had taken me so long. I thanked you for your kindness and said I am okay now and that it was a long time ago. You were about to have your first baby and this news caught me by surprise. I was so happy and relieved you wouldn't have to wait as long as I did to meet your baby.

I had been secretly saving up all my hope for you and you got the positive result we all hoped for your first IVF round. Aren't big sisters supposed to make wishes for their little sisters and have them granted?

We entered a whole new world together and you would soon experience the best job ever, being a mum. I was so happy. Renée shared every scan with the family with pure delight.

Renée showed me a precious ultrasound picture with a pink bow and I could feel myself choking up. The moment I held my niece, Brooklyn, I couldn't hold myself together. I looked at Renée and tears filled my eyes. I know Renée wanted to become a mumma for a long time and to see her with her child was another special sister moment in time. We'd finally both become mothers.

Being the Elvis fan Mum was, she was delighted to have a new grandchild born on Elvis' birthday, 08 January.

I watched as Renée settled in to her new life being a mother. I could see how tired she was and could relate to those first few weeks of being a new mum. Renée always wanted two children, so I knew at some stage she would attempt this world of pregnancies again.

Sometime later Renée called me to let me know she had fallen pregnant again, only this time she didn't need IVF and it was a complete surprise. I was so happy for Renée as I could imagine it feels like a heavy weight being lifted, not needing to go through IVF.

This happiness soon turned to sadness when Renée advised me she'd miscarried. We were all in shock. Renée went from one extreme to the next in a moment, and it was devastating. The world still carries on but a woman losing a pregnancy is a deep brutal hit of pain and it made Renée want to isolate from everyone and everything.

After some time passed, Renée decided if she didn't get her strength to try again, she would never know otherwise. Renée attempted another IVF round and felt incredibly blessed when she got the positive news she was pregnant. I was thrilled as a positive result somewhat changes the path you travel from that moment onwards. It changes from uncertain to certain.

Unfortunately, Renée called me again in tears to let me know that she'd miscarried again and asked me why this was happening. I couldn't answer her. It's a cruel process. When the time was right, I told Renée I believed a miscarriage is a way for the baby to say that something was wrong. We must hold that with as much understanding as possible, to remember with all our heart, but pack it aside safely and gently to put one foot in front of the other and go forward.

That doesn't help a woman who is suffering in the depths of a broken blue heart.

CHAPTER TWENTY-NINE

Two blue hearts

It was a good year later, when Renée attempted another round of IVF without telling anyone, including me. We were so close, but I understand living in the IVF world, you feel like no one can relate and you also want to share the surprise with your support network. Renée doesn't have to tell me everything and later said she couldn't process telling anyone she'd tried and it didn't work (if that was the outcome).

Renée called me at five weeks gestation to advise me she'd completed IVF and not told anyone. She was distressed and said she was pregnant, but feared she was miscarrying again. She immediately rushed to the doctor and had the relevant tests.

The result was what she had hoped for. The baby appeared to be fine, but Renée was incredibly nervous. She knew she was vulnerable because of the last two miscarriages. I chatted to Renée to help her and suggested each pregnancy is a brand new start and like her pregnancy with Brooklyn, this one could just work. I tried to help Renée give this pregnancy the opportunity to be separate from the others.

The days went by and Renée was so sick from morning sickness. She was driving to work with a bucket beside her in case she vomited.

The weeks rolled along, and past the date of both Renée's miscarriages gestation, so this gave her some more hope. Renée asked me if I could please visit her house to mind Brooklyn so she and Adam could go for their twelve-week scan and harmony test. (To check for early pregnancy complications and the baby's gender.)

When Renée and Adam walked back through the door, I knew the baby was okay by the look on their faces. We had a celebration cuddle, and all felt this pregnancy would be just fine. Renée didn't want to tell me the gender for a few minutes. She disappeared, returning with a black balloon and I filmed Renée and Adam popping it to reveal blue confetti. I was just so happy another baby, and this time a baby boy, would join our family.

When Renée started showing, Brooklyn would kiss Renée's tummy to say goodnight to their new baby.

Six weeks later, Renée called Mum and I in tears to let us know she had a scan and her baby would need to be delivered as he was not well. I remember bursting into tears. In one phone call, everything changed. Every time Renée experienced a setback, it opened all my wounds and the torment of thinking it'll be okay and it wasn't.

Brooklyn was rubbing Renée's tummy and asked when the new baby would come out. Renée sat with Brooklyn and said the little baby was sick and wouldn't be staying in Mummy's tummy anymore. Brooklyn immediately got upset and then started laughing at something on the television.

They gave Brooklyn the honorary role of naming this precious little boy. Adam was an avid National Rugby League South Sydney supporter and Brooklyn watched many football games live and on TV. Because of her daddy and his love of football, Brooklyn chose Reggie after the South Sydney rabbit mascot.

Because of Reggie being the 1 in 100,000 chance with his diagnosis, the doctors considered incompatible with life because of the severity. The doctors advised to deliver as there was no other choice. Many days later, after confirming the first scan was correct, Renée and Adam were to attend hospital to deliver their stillborn son, Reggie. Renée said the delivery was excruciatingly painful and incredibly tormenting to deliver a precious baby sleeping, who was so wanted and dearly loved.

Renée and Adam held their boy and spent the day with him in a private room before it was time to say goodbye. Renée said she could hear babies crying in the rooms nearby and this really hurt. Reggie was changed into a sash because the angel outfit was too big for his tiny body. Later that day, it was time for Adam and Renée to say goodbye to Reggie to return home to care for Brooklyn. They placed Reggie in a cold crib and tried to memorise every detail of him before breaking down crying and saying goodbye. Renée said her heart was shattered into irreparable pieces and knew this would traumatise her for life. The funeral director collected Reggie.

Adam and Renée later sat with Brooklyn to explain the little baby was an angel and Brooklyn said she thought he was a star in the sky.

For some time after the doctors delivered Reggie,

Brooklyn kept kissing Renée's tummy to say goodnight to him. Renée said it made her heart ache and made her mummy heart cry uncontrollably.

Our whole family were winded and still are. It just seems so cruel and pointless to lose a child's life in the circumstances Reggie went through. He didn't have a chance to have one day on Earth.

My focus going forward was to encourage Renée to do the basics: eat well, drink water, exercise and sleep. It felt like it was all I could do.

Renée will never be the same. None of us will. Pregnancy for some may be easy. For Renée and I, it was, at times, cruel, painful and absolute bliss.

The most painful part of IVF for me was when it didn't work, after giving your all, you had to somehow step on that unknown path again and into that world of anxiety at every corner. My dear little sister was right there, and it was incredibly hard to witness.

Renée said she now felt what our sister-in-law Rosalie experienced with her son, David. The deaths of their boys united them.

David was delivered by caesarean section at thirty-six weeks and was born with many complications.

One of David's issues was a short gut, which meant that his small intestine failed to absorb food nutrients properly and therefore he couldn't put on weight. David was so malnourished, his bones stuck out and he didn't have bottom cheeks. David couldn't suck properly, so he had a feeding tube inserted into his nose that ran down into his stomach. Rosalie learned to insert the tube herself.

David's biggest battle was a large hole in his beautiful little heart. An Atrioventricular Septal Defect is a hole that encompassed all four chambers of his heart and left David struggling for every breath. Rosalie offered to give David her heart, but the doctors kindly and gently told her that her heart wouldn't fit. This was a battle Rosalie could not help him with.

At two months, specialists attended David to determine whether an operation could save his life. Rosalie was told David was too thin for major heart surgery and because of his short gut, it was unlikely he would ever be strong enough. Rosalie said to be told your child is going to die is devastating because there is nothing you can do. She felt like a failure and like she was dying inside, because there was a beautiful life that she created, and she couldn't fix him.

They then put David in palliative care, and Rosalie commenced watching David die.

When David was three months old, his doctors scheduled a meeting with Rosalie. They told her there is a possibility David might survive surgery by using a special formula that would cause rapid weight gain. Rosalie's hopes soared, and she dared to believe David might come home. Unfortunately, the formula caused fluid to build up in David's lungs. To drain the fluid from his lungs, he needed to come off the formula and subsequently lost any weight he put on.

The darkest day of Rosalie's life came when the doctors informed her that she had two choices. She needed to let David have surgery, which would probably kill him during or after, causing him pain and suffering, or take him off all medications and let him slip peacefully away.

Rosalie knew what choice she needed to make but couldn't fathom how do you make the decision to allow your child to die? How do you sign that piece of paper? With a heavy heart, Rosalie sealed David's fate and she still lives with that guilt and pain. They took David off his medications, and Rosalie prepared to bring him home to die. During what was to be the last few days of his life, he blossomed. His hair grew thick and his size increased, which was unfortunately, just fluid build-up. David had beautiful rosy cheeks. It was like he knew that the struggle would all be over soon.

117 days after David was born, Rosalie, along with her parents, took David for a walk into the hospital gardens. This was the first time he'd ever breathed fresh air. David smelled a flower, listened to the birds sing, and felt the warmth of the sun on his precious face. He seemed happy and peaceful. That evening at 6pm, Rosalie kissed David goodbye and was planning on taking him home the next day.

David slipped quietly away soon after at 7pm. Rosalie received the dreaded call and headed straight back to the hospital and held David and didn't want to let go. David was so cold and Rosalie tried so desperately to warm him up. Rosalie studied his beautiful face for hours, trying to etch memories into her mind. After many hours, Rosalie reluctantly handed her baby back to the Neonatal Intensive Care Unit (NICU) nurses. That was the last time Rosalie ever held her precious David.

They buried David in the beautiful outfit Nanny Lois made for him, Poppy Ian's kilt pin and a toy Peter Rabbit that Poppy bought for him. Rosalie feels she had to leave her baby boy in a cold and dark hole in the ground, which was numbing and heartbreaking.

Rosalie shared with me that when someone you love becomes a memory, that memory becomes priceless. David was a very sick, very frail little boy, but he taught Rosalie the true meaning of strength and unconditional love. Rosalie misses David every day and often wonders what he would be like.

Renée and Rosalie bonded over the loss of their blue hearts and understand each other's pain and wouldn't wish it on anyone. They also look to the stars, like I did, to find some still moments to reflect and find strength.

I have a photo of the sky around the time I was finalising this book. I looked up towards the sky as it was such a beautiful winter's day. The sky was so beautiful and bright blue; however, I noticed an obvious baby shape in the clouds, including a head, eyes, arms, legs, nappy and a torso shaped as a heart. I do wonder which one of the two blue little hearts it was because it was so very clear in that moment. This vision helped me decide on a name for the chapter.

Sometimes visions in the clouds can be interpreted as stories from heaven.

CHAPTER THIRTY

Bedtime story in heaven

At seven weeks gestation, my school friend, Kylie, discovered she was pregnant with twins. In this same moment, Kylie was advised one precious baby had died the week before, being classified as the medical term, non-viable. Kylie was advised the foetus and sac would be absorbed into the placenta and the other twin would continue to grow in its own sac. This provided Kylie with one answer. Because of the separate sacs, they weren't identical. Kylie was advised twin pregnancies are common and most people never know because they don't usually have an ultrasound so early. While coming to terms with losing a twin, Kylie felt extremely grateful the second twin was still with her.

At fifteen weeks' gestation, Kylie had another

ultrasound and knew by the sonographer consulting the doctor that something was wrong. They were concerned there wasn't enough fluid in the sac but couldn't elaborate what it meant. Kylie tried to interpret the accompanying letter to establish a conclusion, however she wasn't able to and would have to wait for clarification from her doctor.

The same afternoon, the doctor was running late for his appointment, so Kylie patiently waited with worry in her heart as she wanted an answer. The doctor read the report and advised he will need to seek an opinion from the professor of foetal care. He explained, as Kylie may have suspected, there were concerns with the baby and explained the baby may have a chromosomal abnormality.

The following week, the professor advised Kylie his concerns were about the head because it was too big and suspected the baby had hydrocephalus (fluid on the brain). At sixteen weeks, it was too early to make a definite diagnosis. The professor opted to conduct a Chorionic Villus Sample (from the placenta), to test for genetic defects instead of amniocentesis (removing amniotic fluid from the sac). Either option could have resulted in a miscarriage. Kylie said she got through thinking of fate. If a miscarriage did not happen, she would take it as a positive sign. If it eventuated, it would be for a reason that something was wrong and she would have to comes to terms with this outcome.

Kylie was advised the results of the sample (chromosomal study) would take two weeks and was warned that even if they come back negative; it doesn't mean everything is okay. It would mean there is no answer yet. The most reliable update would be around 19/20 weeks, which Kylie was advised to be the most accurate time to measure the baby.

The results were negative and Kylie continued to wait for time to pass, while listening to her doctor explain the worst-case scenario, which provided little hope or comfort.

During the painful wait, doctors discovered Kylie had two lumps in her breast, which were later confirmed to be non-cancerous. Kylie continued to focus on her baby and hope her little one is okay. Kylie felt at ease waiting this time and could have waited forever as she was able to keep carrying her baby.

This comfort level was rattled when an ultrasound confirmed that her little boy had hydrocephalus. While he was at twenty weeks' gestation, his head was twenty-two weeks and the fluid was already pressuring his brain. It was unlikely he would make it to full term and if he did, Kylie would have to have a caesarean because the head would be too big for a natural birth. If he survived, he would be severely brain damaged and would not live very long following his birth. Other physical handicaps would not have been known until he was born. Even though the doctors advised he would most likely not live, Kylie considered he might.

The choice came down to inducing the labour or waiting for a premature labour anyway. Kylie couldn't wait for the inevitable, knowing the outcome would never be joyous and she was already mourning the loss of her first twin. There really was no decision to be made. The choice had already been taken out of Kylie's hands.

Kylie was admitted to hospital on 9/9/99 for an induced labour and was given capsules every three hours to make her uterus contract and soften the cervix to encourage dilation. This continued for two days and on the third day, Kylie was placed on a hormonal drip. At 1.54pm, Kylie's baby boy, Brayden, was delivered sleeping, feet first with the cord around his neck, weighing 600 grams and measuring twenty-six centimetres. Brayden had a bilateral cleft palette, which indicated other health concerns. For this reason, the doctor asked for permission for an autopsy, which was granted and would take two months to give an insight into what happened.

Brayden's features mesmerised Kylie and she reflected how much you already love your baby before they are even born. Kylie kissed Brayden and told him how much she loved him. She wrapped him in a blanket made by family and also a love blanket provided by the nurses. Brayden was cold, but Kylie instinctively wanted to protect her son and keep him warm. Kylie didn't want to leave Brayden, she wanted to nurse him back to health.

She felt the tears welling and decided to not say goodbye, which Kylie doesn't regret, because it didn't seem appropriate, given she knew she would see him again. Kylie kissed Brayden on the forehead for the last time and handed him to the nurse as the thought of leaving him alone in his crib was difficult to come to terms with. Brayden's earlier foot and handprints impressions were given to Kylie, along with the love blanket as she wanted something to hold when she left the hospital at 7pm. Kylie knew the longer she stayed, the harder it would be to leave.

When Kylie arrived home, she didn't realise it was going to be so hard. The ache in her heart was unbearable. Kylie wanted her boy back, to hold, love and watch him grow. Kylie went to bed holding the love blanket tight, almost wanting to fill the empty place in her heart. When Kylie was dozing off to sleep, her body continued to breathe the labour pains and she could still hear the midwife saying, 'Big deep breaths, blow out the candle, oooohhhh.' Kylie held the love blanket as tears rolled down her face and onto her pillow with visions of Brayden's perfect little features and double cleft palette. She had a dream the camera which captured Brayden's photos had been ruined.

Kylie was trying to mentally prepare for the visitors and flowers arriving at home. She searched the depths of the cupboards for vases which had been given as gifts and finally realised why she had been given so many. Kylie's body ached, so she lay down and cuddled the love blanket. It became difficult to work out which part of her body ached more, her muscles or her heart.

In the days leading up to the funeral, while making arrangements, Kylie's family were asked if the food was being booked for a party, which brought Kylie to tears. It wasn't an improper question to ask; it was just so emotional for Kylie. It wasn't a party, or a christening, it was for a tiny baby's funeral. Kylie felt she needed to make use of the thoughts in her head and wrote them down in a letter to Brayden.

There were final decisions to make regarding the funeral arrangements, and today she felt more alone than ever as her family returned to work. There were delays with the funeral planning because of the autopsy, which confirmed: a female born at twenty-one weeks, with the narrowing or malformation of the cerebral aqueduct (within the midbrain), leading to ventriculomegaly (enlargement of ventricles of the brain), and the absence of corpus callosum (communication between the two cerebral hemispheres). The autopsy added a whole new layer of grief for Kylie, particularly when she discovered it stated the baby was a girl, when upon delivery Brayden's visual appearance confirmed he was a boy, as did his birth certificate.

During the viewing, which was immediately prior to the funeral service, Kylie's motherly instincts kicked in again, and she made sure Brayden was properly clothed. There were candles, balloons and rose petals around the tiny coffin. On top of the coffin lay a white rose with a blue ribbon. A lullaby played as everyone arrived for the service. The sermon was about angels and Kylie read the letter she prepared a day earlier to Brayden.

At the conclusion of the service, family and friends released balloons in memory of Brayden. Kylie couldn't help but notice two balloons intertwined under the awning where she was standing. Kylie took this as a peaceful sign that her twins were now together and would remain with each other for eternity.

Over the coming weeks, Kylie felt empty. She noticed the flowers people sent had started to wither and die. Kylie wanted to keep some to dry to make pot-pourri, but she couldn't find the energy, because deciding which ones to keep or throw away seemed heartless. Kylie felt this was a parallel to her life. She was putting some flowers in the bin when another fresh bunch was delivered to her door. They were from old friends sending their condolences and she was bracing herself to watch another bunch wither. Kylie had a rosebush in her garden which she'd dedicated to Brayden and it was in full bloom. If only her Brayden could have had the chance to blossom.

Kylie had a picnic day to attend with colleagues and felt out of loyalty to them she should attend, but it was incredibly difficult and she found it hard to concentrate and be present. This was because Kylie felt she had to grieve in silence, because of needing to appear to be strong and focussed for the task at hand. Kylie noted how many weeks into her pregnancy she would be if this harrowing experience never took place. Questions raced through her mind. Would anyone else be taken away from her? How much stronger will she need to be? How much more resilient will she become? How much more can she forgive?

Five weeks passed, and it was Kylie's birthday, which she was dreading. Kylie felt it was too soon for her to be happy about anything, including her birthday. Despite trying, her emotions told her it was difficult to be happy when she was mourning. Some days were good, and some days were bad. It was too early to overcome the grief, but Kylie felt people expect you to get over it, which was incredibly difficult when some people don't understand the ongoing inner torment and process of grief.

Kylie felt it seemed ridiculous, but she was anxious about getting her period again, because she was hopeful she may have already conceived again. She anticipated either outcome would end in tears and reflected how hard it is to believe your heart and soul can be so divided.

Kylie had a new fight on her hands, which was the fight for maternity leave within her employment because of having Brayden's birth acknowledged. Today felt like the launch of an even bigger crusade while maintaining control of her emotions. Kylie pondered that perhaps this is the reason for Brayden's sacrifice, the fight for change.

Eight weeks to the day following Brayden's delivery, Kylie's wave of emotions erupted. Kylie got her period and the crumbling of her insides filled her with inconsolable pain. Her heart was numb and after some time, she surrendered to the hope of 'there will always be next month to try to conceive again.'

Two days later, Kylie took a deep breath as she walked into the office at the cemetery to collect Brayden's ashes. Kylie said it didn't feel right and in hindsight, maybe it was too soon as she just wasn't ready. Concern drove her to collect the ashes when she did because she didn't want them being left at the cemetery for too long. Kylie felt like everyone was watching and knew why she was there, which she felt was absolutely ridiculous to think such a thing. It was as if her soul was laid bare and she carried a sigh stating the obvious.

Not for a second did Kylie think about what other

people were doing there. She felt naked walking in there as if she was fully exposed and getting in and out of there as fast as she could, would mean people would see less.

Kylie scanned the waiting area and noticed various designs on the urns on display and wondered what urn Brayden would be in. The lady at reception advised her someone would be with her in a moment. Kylie was wondering how long this process would take because she wanted to get out of there and reminded herself this was a formality and it needed to happen. Five minutes felt like five hours.

A lady greeted Kylie and welcomed her into her office and offered a seat. She presented Kylie with a white paper carry bag and asked her to check the contents. Auto pilot kicked in and Kylie wasn't really comprehending what was going on around her. Kylie checked the label to confirm it was her Brayden and signed the paperwork. She felt like it was a blur and staying focused meant not crying and therefore losing sense of reality. Kylie's tear ducts were swelling as she carried her boy's ashes outside.

Kylie anxiously examined the contents of the bag. It was a grey plastic box, rectangular, and sealed with wrappings of tape and dollops of blue Silastic. On top was Brayden's plaque from the top of his coffin, which she asked for the day of the funeral and was justifiably denied. Little did Kylie know she would see it again.

The box was relatively heavy and she could hear the ashes sliding around inside, yet hadn't considered what they may look like. Kylie's friend had previously advised her to not be shocked if she found pieces of bone. The visual imagery of dust was hard for Kylie to imagine as she still pictured Brayden's long delicate fingers, broad feet and his gammy little toe. Kylie concentrated on her breathing, knowing she was finally taking her boy home.

Christmas is the time of year when Kylie misses Brayden the most. It's a time of reflection and the first Christmas Kylie remembered how perfect he was. It was hard to believe Brayden was fluttering his little angel wings. Kylie felt she spent this time searching for her lost soul. Her heart still cried and her arms ached to hold her first born and nothing will ever fill that emptiness inside.

During the second Christmas without Brayden, Kylie had a quiet moment reflecting to let him know that this year she had found a little Christmas spirit.

Kylie's strength and courage along with her understanding of things happening for a reason, led Kylie to take the risk of potentially facing more grief and fear by attempting to have more children. She documented her feelings to release her thoughts and emotions. She found the wisdom of accepting she had to try again otherwise she will never know, driven by determination deep within a mother's heart. Kylie drew strength from Brayden and thanked him for his sacrifice, which blessed her with a baby brother for Brayden, named Riley, who was born within twelve months of Brayden's delivery.

She could see the resemblance between her newborn and Brayden and noticed how much bigger Riley was when he was born. Kylie felt when she looked at Riley that he just knew. It was like Brayden and Riley passed each other on the way up and down from heaven. Riley often sat on Brayden's box and pointed to his picture. One of the best moments was when Kylie was feeling sad or thinking about Brayden, Riley would jump into her arms and pat her on the back for comfort.

During Riley's first Christmas, Kylie reflected that Brayden would have most likely been walking. Kylie was sure he would be soaring the heavens and waiting on the staircase to heaven to greet all the other baby angels and one day, his mum.

Time moved on and Kylie had another pregnancy with complications that ended in the loss of her third baby at sixteen weeks' gestation. This pregnancy loss left Kylie living with and rehashing many deep and painful feelings all the while, questioning the mortality and the meaning of existence. This made her want to grab hold of life and tell all the people she loved how important they were.

Kylie had four boys, Riley, Rory, Rhys and Regan and considered them to be blessings to her mother's heart.

After experiencing such grief, Kylie could never imagine feeling such intense joy, and an overwhelming sense of love and fulfilment when she gave birth to each of her boys. Unlike Brayden, her four labours were short. It was like they couldn't wait to get here and didn't want to keep their mum waiting, and likewise Kylie couldn't wait for them to arrive. Kylie's heart overflowed, and she knew her four boys were the true blessings of her life.

The sound of their cries broke the silence of Kylie's grief. Her tears were tears of joy and relief. Where her heart once felt so empty, it was now bursting with love and was so full of hope and expectation for the future. Everything Kylie wanted the world to be finally came true for her, and becoming a mum to four precious boys put her on top of the world.

The connections Kylie feels to her boys and watching them grow brings her a sense of happiness that far outweighs the pain of the past. To love and be loved by her boys is the most precious gift of all. Without the wound in her heart, Kylie says she would never have had an opening to the best and most beautiful part of her life—her four boys.

Kylie has reflected upon her experiences and shares the following insights.

- It strengthens us and we are chosen for the right reasons which may not be revealed at the time.
- We all have a path and are chosen for a reason. Not, Why me? But, Why not me?
- We aren't given anything more in life than we can handle.
- It wasn't her lost babies' time.
- It wasn't meant to be. And even when we try to intervene for the right reasons, there is still a destiny or fate to be fulfilled.

- It is not anything different to somebody else who has gone through trauma.
- We all endure our own versions of pain and tragedy and we survive it.
- The reality could have been far worse than the tragedy.
- As much as it hurts, our babies could have suffered more and we could have suffered too.
- The silent moments are where you must protect your own wellbeing.
- We all have trauma but it is often what we need to put us on our path for us to become who we are meant to be. It gives us courage, strength, compassion, hope, inspiration, belief and even faith.

Kylie knows she has helped so many people with tragedy and death, including people close to her who have spent months in hospital and lost their baby. She views her experiences as part of her journey, to understand grief and help people to heal. Kylie feels she wouldn't have been able to connect, or understand grief, had she have not had her own experiences.

Kylie recently wrote a poem when Brayden would have turned 21. This poem reflects Kylie's own experiences and a bedtime story to read to her firstborn boy in heaven. Kylie feels this poem is Brayden's 21st birthday gift to the world, and dedicates it to parents who don't have the opportunity to read to their babies who were delivered sleeping on earth.

Bedtime Story in Heaven by Kylie Adams

You didn't get a chance to breathe or touch the earth,
I didn't hear you cry at the moment of your birth.
The room was filled with silence and the breaking of my heart,
It was a tragic ending when it should have been the start.

I should have been so hopeful and filled with expectation,
Instead, consumed by grief and lost in contemplation.
Why did this have to happen, why did it have to be?
You were chosen for a reason, even though it's hard to see.

We needed someone strong who could love beyond this earth,
A mother of an angel who would understand their worth.
A special kind of mother who would give you wings

to fly,
    One who has the insight to see reason in the why?

    A selfless love and honour, she will encourage you
to soar,
    Her strength is like no other and comes deep from
within her core.
    Life moves on without you and milestones come
and go,
    Emotions hit like waves and you never really know.

    I can drown in the sorrow or ride the wave to shore,
    Surrender to the feeling and I heal a little more.
    I wonder what you look like, what could have you
achieved,
    But in my heart I feel it, and I can't help but feel
relieved.

    It hurts to be without you, but letting go was for the
best,
    Your wings embrace me from above and leave me
feeling blessed.
    You have made me stronger and more open to
receive,
    Because of you, I have a reason to believe.

    Hope and belief are all some women can hold on

to and even then, it makes you feel vulnerable and question why you might set yourself up for potentially another fall.

"There is a unique pain that comes from preparing a place in your heart for a child that never comes." – David Platt

The pain can be unbearable and consuming and feels like there is no soft landing. The climb back up seems so high and at times unattainable, but this is where outcomes are that can change your life again.

If it is possible, get up one more time than you fall. Renée, Rosalie, Kim, and Kylie all had to believe again after a loss.

Like Rosalie, Kim and Kylie, Renée knew she wanted to hold her little Reggie deep inside her heart and attempt fulfil a desire to have another baby.

Renée's bright little star Reggie was from a fresh cycle of IVF, and there were remaining frozen embryos in storage. Renée hoped if she could bring herself to make the climb back up, there might be a little ray of sunshine sitting in that batch.

CHAPTER THIRTY-ONE

Little Ray of Sunshine in the Shape of a Girl

I never gave birth to a sleeping baby, but I could see the torment within my sister. I knew the miscarriages and loss of Reggie had hit Renée incredibly hard. I wanted to understand more, and I knew she would never be the same. I witnessed a new version of my sister before me. The losses were etched in her heart. I watched her intently to see if there was any way I could assist. I prepared meals, looked after her firstborn, helped with home repairs, made sure she was eating properly and reminded her to look after herself, spiritually, mentally, physically and emotionally.

I don't know how she kept going. Well, I do. It's a mother's heart. It's a powerful force and when we want a child, we find strength we didn't know we possessed.

Renée constantly amazed me. It gave me an insight into how people felt about me, although I couldn't process it because it's just what I did to bring a child into the world.

Time ticks on in a woman's body and Renée was well aware of this. She felt she owed it to Adam, Brooklyn and herself to honour Reggie and get back up.

To our amazement, when Renée still should have been carrying Reggie, she was now pregnant for the fifth time with one living baby. This little baby was from the same batch of embryos as Reggie. This made Renée feel she was close to Reggie for many reasons.

The first trimester was eighty-four days of hope and extreme worry. Would this baby survive? No one could answer this. The twelve-week scan confirmed everything was okay, but so did Reggie's. It was a great milestone to reach, but we were all treading so lightly to help Renée stay as focused as she could be while enjoying the news she really was pregnant again.

The equivalent day Renée gave birth to Reggie passed in this pregnancy and Renée reflected on her little boy. She felt his strength to stay with her for eighteen weeks and asked him for help now to stay strong and she turned his moment into energy for this pregnancy.

Renée reached the halfway mark, and we were all getting a little more comfortable until Renée called from the back of an ambulance at 23.2 weeks while being rushed to hospital. Mum and I broke down when we got the call. Renée was expecting to lose this baby too because we'd all been waiting for the twenty-six week mark as our next milestone. All our research indicated a baby may be okay if born then.

With two miscarriages, one stillborn and serious complications on board in the back of the ambulance, Renée sobbed the whole way to Westmead Hospital. The odds weren't good. Renée called her midwife, who'd helped her through Reggie's pregnancy and was monitoring this one, and she said to Renée to hold on. There could be a glimmer of hope.

Mum and I were at home, and sometimes that glimmer of hope seemed out of reach. It seemed so small compared to all the odds currently against Renée. It was too early in gestation, we imagined, for this baby to survive. But hope is all we had, and we held on with every ounce we had. We cuddled each other and wished for a miracle.

Adam, being the perfect father, cared for Brooklyn at home to keep her routine normal. Brooklyn asked where Mummy was and Adam said she was at the hospital and would be okay.

The same day Renée arrived at the hospital, she called me in a distressed state at 9.30pm. She asked me to please spend the night with her at the hospital as she couldn't be alone. Adam had to be with Brooklyn to settle her to bed.

Jy was asleep by this time and I asked my Mum could she please care for Jy through the night if he needed anything and she did. I asked her to please call me when Jy woke so I could explain to him where I was.

I arrived at the hospital to my see my beautiful little sister and I couldn't stop crying. I did not know if this baby would make it. The grey area for gestation and survival, they informed us, was 24-26 weeks. Renée was currently 23.2 weeks.

Following examinations and tests, Renée was to learn the baby was still on board. I sat beside Renée as she laid in the hospital bed, and I held her hand as I tried to create a positive energy and give Renée somewhere soft to lean. I didn't tell her I was petrified. Absolutely out-of-control petrified. I watched my sister have three pregnancies that did not result in a living child. I felt this could be the fourth. I was out of my element and had no idea how we would manage this going forward.

I encouraged Renée to sleep as I did when I was so worried about my pregnancy as I felt it would calm my body and let my mind rest. Sometimes touch can soothe, and I hoped this contact would bring Renée comfort. I laid beside Renée on the lounge recliner, held her hand, and we both fell asleep. I couldn't get comfortable in the recliner and was sleeping with one eye open in case Renée needed me.

Mum called me as soon as Jy woke that morning and I told him I was okay and was at hospital supporting Aunty Renée and as always, he was compassionate and understanding. I explained Nanny would take Jy to school and I would be there to pick him up, which was possible as Adam would return to spend the days with Renée while Brooklyn was in day care.

I collected Jy from school and asked him if it was okay with him if I were to stay with Aunty Renée again that night in hospital and Nanny would stay with Jy. He understood the whole way through.

I returned to Renée that night, and she still had the baby on board. We sat and pondered what might be. Mum gave Renée a pot plant with a stone that read 'Hope'. Renée told me that a lady, like her, was placed on full bed rest and lasted fifteen weeks. If this happened to Renée, she would be thirty-nine weeks pregnant. This was a glimmer of hope we needed to cling on to. Under the weight of dark clouds, we were hoping for a little ray of sunshine.

As Renée was on complete bed rest, I didn't want her to have to roll over in the night to press the buzzer if she needed help. To me, complete bed rest is just that. I stayed with her and pressed the buzzer whenever she needed assistance. I also went to Oporto to get Renée her favourite take away meal.

Every day this baby stayed on board brought us hope. I made Renée a sign and placed in on the cupboard directly across her bed. It had a big twenty-seven on it. This was the week of gestation, which I was trying to help Renée focus on. I planned to change this sign every week.

On a Thursday night, nine days after they admitted

Renée to full bed rest, she told me she had bad lower back pain. She was tossing and turning through the night and I was helping as much as I could. This continued through Friday.

We woke on Saturday morning and Renée asked for an ultrasound as she needed to hear her baby's heartbeat. My heart was racing when the first nurse couldn't find a heartbeat and called for a senior nurse. I looked at Renée and we didn't say anything but I'd seen her sad eyes so many times before and was keeping a lid on my tears because I just couldn't break down now. The second nurse appeared, and the air was tense. The nurse tried to find this baby's heartbeat and after a few attempts, finally did. Phew! I took a photo of Renée as this scan happened. I didn't know that it would be the last photo Renée would have of her being pregnant.

They'd planned that Adam was coming in to spend some time with Renée this same morning, before returning home to care for Brooklyn. We'd arranged that this would coincide with a Saturday soccer game for Jy. Renée's gestation was 24.6 weeks and I would be gone for three hours. Adam arrived, we tagged our care of Renée and never left her without support. I said goodbye to Adam and Renée and said that I will be back soon.

I was watching Jy play soccer when my phone rang. It was Adam. He said they'd moved Renée to the delivery room as a precaution following this morning's ultrasound, which I was present at. He then rang me back soon after to advise me the baby was about to be born.

I burst into tears. Last time Renée gave birth, her baby was born sleeping. I knew well from years of IVF training you give grace to each pregnancy to allow it to form into its own experience. I was holding onto my trained mindset in this moment but couldn't hold back the tears. Renée and Adam gracefully accepted if the journey for this baby was too hard, they couldn't expect their unborn baby to struggle and live with pain and suffering and would have to accept what they were dealt. I quietly hoped for a miracle.

I desperately wanted to be with Renée and Adam, but this was their moment and they didn't know what lay ahead. My boy was proud to have me watching him on the soccer sidelines. Little did he know what was happening in this moment in time.

To this point, Mum had conducted over thirty years of voluntary street ministry. She was on duty when I called to let her know about the baby. We both cried and cried.

After Jy's soccer game, I sat with Mum as we waited for Adam's call to let us know how the delivery went. My phone rang. It was Adam, and I braced myself.

He said, "Hi Jodi, the baby is alive. She weighed 650 grams, was 29.5cms in length and was placed on a breathing machine. Renée is okay."

Mum and I cried again. We knew for this little precious girl to survive, it would be a long road ahead, but hope is what you must have. Because sometimes the sun shines through.

A lady was running a crystal stall nearby and noticed Mum and I crying and came over with an angel crystal to offer her support and strength to our family. We continued to receive updates throughout the day and the baby was still with us. In honour of her mum, they named this precious little girl Bonnie Renée.

I was on my way back to spend the night with Renée and I could see as I was passing the delivery suites there was a film crew in the hospital filming the Australian series, One Born Every Minute. I arrived at Renée's room and gave her a massive cuddle. She looked so sad, worried and was in pain from the delivery and broke down crying. Renée told me she'd just got back from seeing Bonnie for the first time, some ten hours later. She was so tiny, and she worried about her.

I spent that night and the following four nights with Renée in the maternity ward. The nurse from the NICU brought in Bonnie's first photo. Renée and I couldn't stop staring at Bonnie's picture and hoping she would be okay. I placed Bonnie's photo near the plant and hope rock Mum bought Renée and we kept sending all our energy to Bonnie.

I was reading success stories on the wall of the NICU unit but was concerned because Bonnie was so young and there weren't that many stories with babies born at 24.6 weeks. Would Bonnie survive? We wouldn't get this answer.

When Bonnie was four days old, they discharged Renée from hospital. I took a photo of Renée dressed and ready to leave hospital holding a photo of her baby and I was crying on the inside. I couldn't let on how sad I was as Renée was struggling enough. All Renée could do was hope she could soon bring Bonnie home too.

I needed to take something to Bonnie but could only chat to the nurse in the reception area of NICU because of strict medical protocols of only Mum and Dad being allowed to see Bonnie. It would be many more weeks before I could meet her.

After the first week, Bonnie contracted an infection and was fighting for her life. Her survival rate was 60%. They diagnosed Bonnie with a dislocated right shoulder (from delivery), a patent ductus arteriosus in her heart, a grade 1-2 brain bleed on her brain, highly underdeveloped lungs and couldn't tolerate milk. The outlook was grim.

Bonnie got through her first week and surprised the medical team. She had an undeniable strength and desire to fight.

By the second to third week, there became some scary signs Bonnie had developed a life-threatening infection in her bowel. They placed her on strong antibiotics and our family waited, hoped and prayed she would not leave us.

After ten gruelling days, it became apparent Bonnie would need surgery on her bowel. They rushed her over to Westmead Children's Hospital and performed surgery within hours. Bonnie was okay but lost eighteen centimetres of her bowel. This was because of the infection and internal hernia that wrapped around her bowel.

The next two weeks were so nice until the nightmare bowel infection returned. They took Bonnie back to the Westmead Children's Hospital and performed further surgery. It turned out to be curdled milk blocking Bonnie's bowel.

Once Bonnie overcame her major obstacles, she was allowed to have visitors. Renée invited Mum and I to meet Bonnie. We went into the nursery separately because of medical standards to protect the little ones. What a sight she was. She had a pretty little face, just like her big sister Brooklyn. She looked warm and was feeding, which was a great sign. Renée separately explained to Mum and I how the machines worked and what Bonnie's readings were. I got a beautiful photo with Bonnie beside her crib and my eyes were red from crying happy tears.

On the same day I was allowed to meet Bonnie, Kate Ritchie (Australian actress, radio presenter and children's author), was visiting the ward Bonnie was in.

Kate spoke to Renée about Bonnie. Renée shared how brave Bonnie was. Kate listened intently to Bonnie's story and wished for a wonderful outcome.

Renée said she was feeling the impact of being in hospital for so long and a bit disconnected from the world outside the hospital. Kate's conversation was a welcome distraction and Renée said she was delightful and has a very kind, caring and beautiful soul.

Bonnie spent ninety-six days in hospital and came home at 38.5 weeks. She received almost five hundred lots of medication, twelve cannulas, two peripherally inserted central catheters, two regular catheters, eleven blood transfusions, six eye examinations, several tummy ultrasounds, many x-rays, six weekly vaccinations, countless poking and probing. In true Bonnie spirit, she hardly ever complained. The early photos are private and heartbreaking.

I bought Bonnie a doll and Bonnie wore this doll's clothes as she was too small for six zero baby clothes. I wanted to give Bonnie this gift so she can dress her doll one day in the clothes she wore in her first few months of her life.

Renée later asked me to be Bonnie's godmother,

which is a real honour as I feel like I slept beside Bonnie for twelve nights while she was in her mummy's tummy on bedrest and when we were separated following Bonnie's birth as she was being meticulously cared for in NICU. Bonnie and I go way back!

I credit Renée and the medical team for saving Bonnie's life. Renée stayed on bed rest for as long as she could. Bonnie fought as hard as she could and the doctors and nurses from NICU Westmead and Grace Centre at Westmead Children's Hospital were so wonderful, caring, professional and helped nurse Bonnie to good health. Adam was a magnificent support to Renée and kept his family at the forefront of all decisions he made.

I heard my little sister cry tears of extreme worry and concern when I laid beside her in hospital while holding her hand. We longed to hear a heartbeat at every ultrasound.

When the dark clouds and storms are about, it is in these times that if we can push through, the little ray of sunshine appears. Renée's little ray of sunshine in the shape of a girl named Bonnie reminds Renée of her twin IVF brother Reggie, who appears in the stars in the sky every night. Reggie guides Renée. He gave

Bonnie strength. He guides us all.

Bonnie, like the pot plant which Mum bought, is thriving. Bonnie has just turned one. For her first birthday, I bought her an engraved brooch with a blue bird as a sentimental gift, similar to what my beautiful mum bought me as a little girl. Yesterday when I had lunch with her, she held onto my hands and started to walk. Bonnie has the brightest smile every time I see her and I look back at her with so much admiration. She truly amazes me. I will forever be in awe of the courage Bonnie showed. Little does she know how many lives she has touched. In the words of Bonnie's Doctor "Bonnie's story is one of science and a fairy tale." Bonnie is my inspiration and is the definition of bravery, strength and courage.

Soon after Renée settled Bonnie in her new environment at home, she wanted to find a way to bring happiness to children.

Renée commenced a balloon business, BBBBalloons (BBBBalloons Facebook, bbbballoons Instagram, Renee Kaida YouTube), creating unique displays and online tutorials to share the steps involved.

This endeavour would prove to be very therapeutic

and healing for Renée.

I'm incredibly proud of my Little Sister for getting back up again and wanting to help people smile, particularly children.

CHAPTER THIRTY-TWO

Thank Goodness for IVF

At times I have an old soul and have often said I should have been born generations ago but having said that, I'm grateful for everything the modern age offers.

If I was born in my grandmother or mother's era, I wouldn't have a child. For this reason, I was in awe of the science behind my IVF journey every step of the way. This gift of IVF gave me a child who changed my world.

I felt at a loss, yet comfortable and was certain I was with the right IVF medical team, by the confidence displayed by my Fertility Specialist and my Obstetrician, Dr Jyotica Ruba. I had all hope riding on their choices and they made me feel comforted and safe in their care.

Our doctors and nurses are the most magical people. I'm sure they know it, but from one lady who was in awe of what you did and how you looked after me, I say thank you from the bottom of my heart. The professionalism, care and interest displayed made me feel like I was the only patient. I had to keep turning up. You did your job, and I did mine.

There were ten rounds of IVF where it didn't work for me and I knew I needed to get back up (again). I endured: eighteen operations/sedations, eight completed IVF cycles with negative pregnancy results, two cancelled cycles (one due to overstimulation from the hormone injections, the other because the eggs didn't fertilise into embryos). Also, one hundred and fifty blood tests, nine hundred needles in my stomach including all the IVF injections, daily blood clotting prevention needle (every day of my pregnancy in my stomach), four insulin needles a day in my stomach (for the last nine weeks of my pregnancy) and many daily diabetes finger blood checks. Along with numerous ultrasounds, considerable expense and no guarantee (ever) that it would work.

I needed to survive the heartache. I needed to sink

or swim and I swam for a child I dreamt of to have a chance at life. I fought for my mummy heart. I turned thoughts of total despair into opportunities to think positively. I sat isolated and found a way to continue. I was brave and faced my fear of needles. Even though I needed a break and wanted to give up, if I stopped, it was all over. I needed to keep going.

This journey has changed my life forever. I still feel the pain of waiting. Ten unsuccessful IVF attempts over almost three years is a lot of anxiety, distress and grief before success. I am a different person now because of this. It doesn't end when you have a baby. The sustained and repeated trauma is not something you easily forget. So many things about failed IVF rounds are triggered for me every day, but it's in the distance and manageable.

There were many winding roads and heartrending moments, lots of tears (both happy and sad). I had a tremendous support network, a strong mind, a fight to fulfil a mother's heart, a positive pregnancy result and one strong baby boy. I gave it all I had to become a mother.

Thank you for the gift of science and our brilliant dedicated professionals in the medical world who make our dreams come true. This is particularly the case with Renée, Rosalie, Kim, Kylie and myself. We are so grateful.

CHAPTER THIRTY-THREE

Thank you to my flame - my miracle baby named Jy

To my dear miracle child, my Jy Jy (nickname), after many years, I was waiting in the delivery room and listening intently for a baby's cry and then I heard you. I just got shivers typing this. This moment of elation and triumph is forever etched in my mind and will forever be one of my favourite moments.

I love you with all my heart. You are my miracle, and I still can't believe after all the heartache, my son, that you are here. I have accepted that maybe your mummy will forever be in amazement of what we achieved.

Thank you for:

- being the flame I could feel in my heart,
- revealing why I couldn't stop trying,
- bringing my dream to life,
- your kindness,
- holding my hand,
- the songs you sing to me,
- the sweet words you say to me,
- bringing me so much love, peace and joy that only you can bring,
- teaching me patience, unconditional love and sheer determination.

You're ten now and you have changed my life and I love you so much. I blossomed in a whole new way when you entered my life. Mummy wants to finally get a puppy for us to care for. I am settled, thanks to you, my boy.

Together with your pet rabbit, Pee Wee, and your new puppy, Scooby Doo, I can foresee us having years of fun and laughter caring for these two beautiful pets.

You never cease to amaze me, Jy. You recently came home from school with 'I love you Mum' written on your arm and school shirt and you asked me to never wash the shirt. You are the most loving boy and I'm so incredibly moved by the connection we share. I'll tuck your shirt away in a safe spot for you, sweetheart.

When we recently sat and watched your birth video together, I watched the amazement in your face. You thought it was so spectacular to watch yourself being born and talked to your younger self on the screen and said, "You can do it Jy." You sure can my boy. You said I was so sweet when I was crying happy tears after holding you for the first time. How sweet they were.

I still can't believe I can touch you and you are real. You are the greatest gift I've ever received. I'm so incredibly blessed.

I love watching you play soccer, particularly goal keeper because you are so skilful. You have the funniest sense of humour and constantly make me laugh.

I love your dance moves and singing when you decide you want to put on a performance for Nan and me. Your musical talent is so impressive. My favourite video of you is your medley of Thunderstruck (ACDC), Viva Las Vegas (Elvis Presley) and Saturday Night (Cold Chisel) on the ukulele.

You have always been kind to babies and animals, and I feel this is an insight into your true character.

Don't ever change these qualities Jy, as they will take you a long way in life. Promise me to always believe in yourself because that's where the magic is.

With an educated decision, stand up for what you believe in, even if that means standing alone.

I want you to find a way to forever be determined in life. Just like I was in bringing you to life.

I wrote this story to inspire people all around the world, and for you, Jy. I wanted to document this chapter in my life so you can understand what I did to become a mother and how much I wanted you. I hope you enjoy this story and always remember I love you dearly.

You are so loyal and supportive and I'm incredibly proud to call you my son.

I am proud of you, both now and what you achieve in the future.

'There are two things we should give our children; one is roots and the other is wings.' — W. Hodding Carter.

My mummy heart will always be by your side, no matter where you fly.

It's now time to help others with our story.
Seek and you shall find.

I know I did my best.

I DID IT!

We did it, my little heart.

We are a great team.

I created a precious life.

I carried this precious life for 270 days and in my heart forever.

An IVF Miracle from Mahers.

Miracles really do happen.

His name is Jy.

Signed by Jy.

Jy

Thank You

Thank you to you, the reader, for allowing me to tell you my story. I wish in some way that my guests' stories and my journey have helped to connect, shine a ray of hope or inspired you and/or people you care about.

To all the people in the world who are trying to face and conquer a difficult infertility, IVF process or assisted conception and everything that comes with a pregnancy and/or loss, I wish you all the very best and please look after yourself and each other. I can guarantee you that you are in not in this alone.

To all the people who have achieved their babies through so much suffering, my heart goes out to you and I commend you for what you have been through and conquered. I hope you are okay. I wish you all the best and want you to know that you didn't go through this alone.

To all the Dietitians, Naturopaths and Counselllors who study to assist people through the utmost of difficult times, thank you so much for your care and professional guidance.

To the organisations who coordinate and foster parents who adopt children, thank you so very much for being angels on earth and looking after these children and their families. I'm in constant awe of your kindness and deep powerful desire to make the world a better place for children.

To Lauren, thank you for introducing me to Karen from my publishing company, White Light Publishing. Karen, thank you for our first phone call when you believed in me and my story. It was a defining moment for you to agree to work with and support me to sprinkle my story all around the world. You are an inspiration yourself. Well done, Karen. To Dannielle, thank you for our chats and your encouragement throughout the editing process. We sure did connect over the topic of pregnancy. You independently confirmed for me that this book will help people. You are both extraordinarily talented women, and authors yourselves, and I'm absolutely thrilled that both of you wonderful ladies helped me bring this book to life. To Dylan and Chelsea, thank you for assisting me with so many changes to my book. You kindly accepted my ideas with professionalism and helped to produce a book I'm so incredibly proud of. You have all been amazing to work with and came highly recommended by another author of yours, my friend, Greg Bridge, who published Yes, Health Matters in the Workplace.

Thank you, Greg, for your courage and inspiration with your book and guiding me to the best publishing company in the world. Continue to pursue the amazing work you thrive at, which is helping people in their personal and professional lives.

A heartfelt thank you to my dear Mum Cheryl, Dad

Allan, Brother Ian, Sister Renée, extended family and close friends for their unrelenting support. You offered me somewhere soft to fall as I travelled down one of my toughest roads to become a mother. Thank you, my rock solid family.

Thank you to Mum and Renée for taking so many telephone calls of my despair. I tried to hold some anguish in because I knew you were suffering too, but you encouraged me to let it all out. Thank you for holding me tight and helping me find the courage to keep focused by advising me to 'take one day at a time'. When I was really shattered and had lost all hope, these words somehow gave me a reason through all the darkness. To see the light at the end of the tunnel, even if that tunnel only lasted until the next medical step.

Mum, I recall you growing up saying, "We all have adversity, it's how we handle it." This was one of my biggest challenges, and I handled it as best as I could. You are the best mother a child could ever want. I am so lucky, Mum. You have been absolutely amazing to me and I will never forget. The definition of a mother is you. Loving, caring, supportive, persistent, patient and unfaltering support. I look forward to the next chapter of our lives with a big smile and a warm heart. Meet you for a hot chocolate at Beale Street, Mumma Bear. xo

Dad, I remember us talking about grandchildren and I could see the delight and hope in your eyes. I really tried Dad before you fell asleep forever, but I just couldn't make it happen any sooner. I know you don't want me to say this, but I am sorry I couldn't give you a grandchild to hold before you left us. It stings me, but I know you don't want me to suffer, so I have accepted this is life. While I kept powering forward through IVF, I never forgot your words, 'No Maher ever gives up.' I struggled after you passed away dad, but your spirit, you coming to me in my dreams and your love and support kept me going and will continue to do so. You never met my little bundle of joy, but please know I cried tears of joy for both you and me when Jy was born, as I'd been graced with the baby we often talked about. We talk about you all the time. Jy often speaks of you when I am putting him to bed. He has asked me how you died and often pretends he is you when he is encouraging and supporting me. He said he doesn't want me to have a heart attack and wants me to be on planet Earth for one thousand years. Your spirit lives on in your grandson, Dad. He is just like you. He is happy, has a great sense of humour and is a fighter. I have been given the precious gift in this little boy. Thank you for helping to encourage, guide and love me. I will raise a wonderful young man. Until we meet again, Dad.

Thank you to Ian, Rosalie, Allan, Charlee, Wyatt, Adam, Renée, Brooklyn, Bonnie, Aunty Kathy, Uncle Norris, Aunty Janelle, Vickie, Daniel, Shane, Sarah, Jarryd, Blake, Ian, Lois, Lynne, the Dawson, Kaida, Maher, Marsden, Nicholson, Russell, and Townsend family. Along with Uncle John, Nanny Jessie, David, Reggie, Robyn, Peter and Maxie who are resting peacefully. It takes a village to raise a child, so thank you all for inspiring and helping Jy and me.

Thank you to Amanda, Amy, Cathy, Dana, Emma, Peita, Peta-Jade and my special editing friend for just being there. You truly are great friends and helped me push through every time IVF didn't work. When things fall apart, friends keep it together. Thank you. x

Thank you to the IVF medical world, your gift is truly amazing, and it makes me feel fortunate to have been born in an era where the brilliance of science has made me a mother. Many brilliant people who have passed away, have contributed to the science we are fortunate to have access to today. Science and fairy tales are what I wish for every medical patient. Thank you for your support right across the world.

Thank you to my dear little sister Renée and her husband Adam, for calling me that night in utter shock about two little lines on that first pregnancy test stick. I felt like I needed to convince you both you were pregnant and I still smile that I was part of that precious moment with you both. It was touching to listen to the happy shock in both your voices. Thank you, Adam, for being a wonderful support.

Dear little sister Renée, your journey was as painful as mine. You had so many results. Your three beautiful children are a testament to your flame inside you to be a mummy. It was dark and difficult for so long and I'm so honoured you are my sister. Reggie shines brightly in the night sky. You became a living story, like the IVF story I read that continually inspired me. I constantly look at you in awe of what you pushed through and the family you created. This is all here because you were brave enough to get back up again and again. You did it! I did it! We did it, sister! May your babies forever guide you and rest in peace little Reggie xo

When Brooklyn was four, she was talking to Mum on the phone and asked her when she was going to heaven to dance with Reggie. Mum said to Brooklyn that it was beautiful for her to speak of Reggie being so happy. Thank you Brooklyn, for keeping your heavenly little brother's spirit alive in our family xo

Dear Rosalie, I believe your little boy David's spirit gives you courage and determination to succeed in all aspects of your life. You're very special. He wouldn't want you to be tormented and in pain. You did what any loving mother would do to help prolong his life, along with making the difficult and selfless decision for his suffering to stop. I feel David's story will connect to people who share/d the same outcome. It was my honour to relay your precious boy's story so he can live on. I promise you David is not forgotten. Fly high and inspire many, you precious little boy. May your babies forever guide you and rest in peace David xo

Dear Ian, Rosalie and family, thank you for your kind words and encouragement, especially throughout IVF. I'd be lost without you both. I can't say it any other way. Thank you from the bottom of my heart for throwing me a lifeline. Your beautiful earth children, Allan, Charlee and Wyatt make my heart sing. I just love them. I'm the proudest aunty. Looking forward to many more years together with our children. xo

Music has played a significant role in my life. My brother, Ian, is the music man in our family and often says, "Sis, you've got to listen to this one." After Jy was born, Ian took me aside and said he had to play a song for me. I knew by the look on his face he'd found another great song. Ian turned it up really loud and we were playing our air guitars and rocking around the loungeroom.

It took me some time to let go of the hold IVF had on my life as it had become a deep engrained mode of finding ways to be consistently strong and tested my endurance every day. Certain songs made me realise how far I'd come and gave me a nudge to return to me, to who I was before IVF. I tried to let go and release the heartache from the IVF turmoil that shaped the day-to-day person I'd become. I didn't feel I would ever forget the torment and heartbreak, but I'd stepped onto another path with a little person who I was responsible for. I feel a sense of a massive accomplishment every time I hear powerful songs. Thank you, Ian and Rosalie, for helping me through with music.

Dear Kim, when I first heard your story, I couldn't process the enormity of what you went through to create your family. We didn't know each other when we went through our tough moments to create our children. It's been a blessing to meet and help inspire each other. Particularly when our tears fall while we speak of our heartache and triumph. These precious little babies we have are a testament to our fight and will to not give up. To all your babies in heaven, your mum is an angel on earth and has many friends who will catch her tears and also make her smile. Your earth family talk of you all the time and feel your spirit. I can promise you all, that we will take care of your mum Kim, dad Damien, brothers and sister: Zachary, Scarlett, Lachlan and William who light up your parents' lives. Stay safe and warm with Poppy. (This helps your mummy feel peace.) May your babies forever guide you and rest in peace xo

Remember the night you were proofreading your two chapters? I couldn't stop laughing and crying with you from a distance. You texted me from your bathroom across town, which is where you could grab a few moments. You said you burst into tears how the story we worked on together connected emotionally with you and captured your journey perfectly. Then your children noticed you were missing and snuck fingers under the door and started knocking as they wanted their mum. You quickly wiped your tears because you didn't want your children to wonder why you were crying. They will find out when they read this.

Dear Kylie, your Mum Maureen, who is now in heaven, was our netball coach while we were at school. I had a thought a few days ago and relived phoning her to tell her that I didn't want to play netball anymore. I felt I was letting her down. This flashback was around the time you posted acknowledging Brayden's 21st birthday. I couldn't help but contact to send you support and love. You advised me that you had written Brayden a poem for his birthday. I was due to send my book to the editor for the final time and couldn't let it go without seeking your permission to include your very moving poem.

It sure was a divine intervention. On our final day of reviewing your chapter, you were celebrating Rory's 18th birthday. This made me smile. Your boys, like my boy, are forever making you happy and from a dear old friend, it's beautiful to see your mummy heart smile. Thank you for the beautiful gift you have of guiding, educating and helping people. Your real life experiences make you truly understand what grief is and we are all incredibly blessed by your kindness, warmth, spirit and ability to get back up. May your angels forever guide you and rest in peace xx

Thank you to the lady I had the light bulb moment with to write this book. I considered writing my story for the first five years of Jy's life, but it just didn't seem like the right time. That was until a chance encounter with a lady I'd just met. We got talking about children and I shared my IVF journey. This particular lady, Susanna, was amazed and got shivers when I told her my story as she did my hair for my sister's wedding. I mentioned I'd considered writing a book about my IVF story. Susanna asked me to promise her I would write the book and tell the world my story. I looked her in the eye and said, "Okay, I promise I will write my story." It was now out there, and I honoured my word. Thank you so much Susanna for seeing something in me, for putting me on the spot and making me commit to you I would write this book.

The feedback I received in the review stage of this book was touching. I received a hand-written note from a woman in her 70s who said she didn't read a lot but was moved by my story. She thanked me for explaining how difficult and rewarding my journey was. She explained this medical assistance wasn't around when she had children and my journey intrigued her. I also received a wonderful email from a family friend of over fifty years, Maureen. She explained I made her cry, but it was a relief as it let out some of her fertility pain she'd been holding onto for four decades. Thank you to my circle of family and friends who helped me bring this book to life. I am so proud of our team effort.

Thank you to Angela G for successfully taking over my job during maternity leave. Little did we know that would lead us to letting our creativity flow together (in that place). When I first approached you to surprise you with the only page I'd written of this book, which was the cover, you surprised me.

You said, "I talk to people about you all the time. Now I can give them your book."

I must admit, I didn't know what to say and was flattered. Thank you for this compliment and for believing in me that day. I often shared with you how many words I'd written, knowing I was aiming for a particular word count to finish my book. I couldn't wait to tell you each time I'd typed more. It was a delightful milestone we reached together, typing the last word of this book as we listened to 'Somewhere Over the Rainbow'. Thank you for preparing me a congratulatory afternoon tea to mark the occasion. I enjoyed sitting in the glorious sunshine in those bright yellow seats as nature's confetti fell from the tree above us. Your banana and chocolate cake was scrumptious and is now my favourite. Thank you immensely for your beautiful soul and the hours you have graciously given perfecting this book for me. There will always be rainbows in our life.

Thank you to Emma for inviting me to join you for a spectacular night on Sydney Harbour as we enjoyed chocolates overlooking the breathtaking sights Sydney offers while we reviewed the final version of this book. I found out six years on how difficult it was for you to have two pregnancies in front of me as I went through IVF. I thought of you and how this may have been for you along the way. I didn't let my sadness show when you were pregnant as I made a promise to myself that you deserve me supporting you as I would if I weren't trying to get pregnant. I called you three days after the birth of your second child to advise you I was pregnant. You were just about to leave hospital and I can't repeat what you said as I'd need to censor it!. That call for me was pure delight. I was so proud of us both. You were with me throughout this whole IVF journey. Thank you for pushing me, for giving me medical information, for never letting me give up and for my new skincare range that you snuck in my bag after this wonderful weekend together.

Thank you to Peita for constantly reminding me about my dad and how proud he would have been of me. I felt like quitting sometimes, but you made it simple for me to take a breath, have a rest and try again. I remember telling you how down and out I was, and I knew I could lean on you to pull me through, to stand again emotionally and try again. I remember waiting in the room for you when you had your son, and I was overwhelmed for you. It would be many years on that you offered me support that helped me cross the IVF finish line.

Thank you to my local support network: Allan, Bellinda, Carolyn, Christina, Heather, Hedy, Jan, Kelly, Kim, Kristy, Kym, Lisa, Mel, Marissa, Sharon and Simone. Your constant every day support and input with ideas about my book cover helped me tremendously, particularly at the 11th hour. I changed it a few times and I'm thrilled with the final version. The colours make me feel calm. Bellinda so kindly helped me with her artistic flair and also taught Jy to paint a bright beautiful koala. It proudly hangs on my wall at home and was the inspiration for the colours of my book cover. Thank you all for your friendship and support for Jy and me.

Bellinda, you may recall a discussion about influencing children by conducting art classes. How about we ask everyone that reads this book to take out the blank canvas, paint, crayons, textas and pencils and ask their children to do art every week. They can make wall art, posters, gift wrap and art books to encourage children to weave so much colour and texture into their life. I know it means the world to you for art to make a difference and you believe that art truly does heal and changes lives. Being an art lover myself, here is a world stage to share your message. You're welcome.

To my local network of Teachers and Educators, thank you from the bottom of my heart for reaching not only my son, but all the children who blossom from your guidance and passion which leads to influencing children in ways that change their lives.

Quoting Bellinda's words, "Students are curious, intrigued, feel compelled, enthusiastic, and passionate about learning, inquiring, and mastering. They have not only an "I CAN" attitude, but also an "I ENJOY" feeling. These habits of thinking are hallmarks of successful, intelligent thinkers."

A dear friend from school, Tracy and I had remained in contact and empowered and inspired each other throughout life. I noticed Tracy wearing a beautiful floral, teal colour dress and messaged her to compliment her choice of dress. I didn't know, but Tracy then purchased me the same dress and contacted Mum to arrange a surprise delivery. You have a beautiful soul. As you are a Children's Educator, we are so lucky to have people like you care for our babies we fight so hard to get.

Dear Deborah Knight, I watched you on television. I honestly don't know how you were present in a public role that demanded such dedication and commitment when I knew what you would be going through medically to have one baby. I could see the schedule you were committed to and the 'mask' you were wearing. I suspected your mummy heart would be hurting. I don't know how you did it, day after day, particularly following negative pregnancy results. Your mummy heart was as focused as mine was. We both dug so deep for strength. I praise your dedication to undertake IVF as often as you

did, and I'm so genuinely happy for you because you're
a delightful person and deserved a positive result from
sheer determination. My worried heart for
you turned into happiness. From one IVF mum to
another, with twenty-three rounds of IVF between us
– congratulations. We did it!

Karen interviewed me for my book launch on Dad's
birthday 27th November 2020. He would have been so
proud of me launching my book on his birthday.

Before the final print run of my book, I met a lady
named Charisse. This beautiful lady before me was very
interested in my story.

Charisse advised me she was so pleased she found
me and my book and apologised for being an emotional
mess. Charisse mentioned she didn't realise her ten
rounds of IVF was still so raw. It's not a topic Charisse
says she discusses often as it does not come up in general
conversation, and she feels it is a hidden struggle.

Charisse thanked me immensely for writing my book
so others can understand our journey.

Charisse later mentioned she hoped I don't mind her
saying 'our story', even though I wrote my book, as she felt
our journey is so similar.

I wrote my book to inspire many people including
people like Charisse who have suffered through IVF as
much as we have.

I commend you on your determination Charisse and will never forget your raw emotion and gratitude as we discussed 'our story' xx

To my dear fertility specialist, who I visited from my second round of IVF and beyond; you gave me so much comfort by confidently suggesting the next approach. I was disheartened walking into your clinic after an unsuccessful attempt, but I always left with more hope because of you. I thank you from the bottom of my heart for nurturing me to believe we can do this again. For helping me, for not giving up on me and providing me such comforting words when I was down and out. I placed my trust in you and leaned on your professional skills to get me through. I remember your compassion and devastation when my attempts did not result in a pregnancy. You went above and beyond to help me and that carried me to the next round. You took a photo of my embryos up on the television screen and delightedly handed me my first picture of my baby. I thank you so very much for your care and dedication to help devastated people, like I was, turn their life in a completely different direction. You have such a critical role in the process for an IVF patient, one that you excel at. You are simply amazing. Keep spreading your magic because you make people like me very happy. You weave miracles into people's lives and I will never forget you.

Dear Jy's Paediatrician, when Jy was on the resuscitation table, I really thought I was losing him but your support and diligence, I believe, was where the big decisions were made that helped to keep my boy earth side. Thank you for your care, support and constant contact to let me know of Jy's progress. I leaned on your confidence and dared to believe that Jy would be okay. Your care and constant monitoring of Jy until he was eighteen months old is gratefully appreciated. Thank you for your passion to care for all children and their families. You weave miracles into people's lives and I will never forget you.

Dear Dr Jyotica Ruba, I felt an instant rapport with you and that made me feel free and excited. I knew I would be in good hands with you. I remember laying on the bed as you prepared me for my seventeen-week scan and you told one very excited Mummy-to-be that she was having a boy! Your compassion, care, beautiful manner and experience comforted me throughout my pregnancy. When I was anxious for positive updates about Jy during each scan, I believed and trusted you which helped me settle. You kept your word to deliver on the agreed date, so I didn't have to embroid Jy a new suit! What a good sport you are! Hearing the delight in your voice as you wished Jy a happy birthday when you lifted him in the air towards me, makes me still cry tears of happiness to this day. It was such a breathtaking moment. Once Jy was in your hands, I knew you would protect him until he was medically cleared to meet his mummy. Thank you for looking after Jy and me and making sure we were both safe throughout the delivery.

You have such a critical role in bringing a child into the world, and I watched you work with confidence. Your manner comforted me, and I was so relieved to know I had the most brilliant obstetrician right beside me. You are a true professional who weaves miracles into people's lives and I will never forget you. I didn't know when I met you that you would inspire the spelling of Jy's name.

Thank you to my previous employer for allowing and supporting me to be absent from work utilising my sickness leave, while I made this miracle come to life. Thank you for recognising the valuable role women play when creating children, the significant role they play by raising them and by supporting maternity leave and return to work policies.

Thank you all my family and friends for your love, unwavering support and moving mountains to help me raise my miracle. Jy and I will forever be grateful.

And lastly, no matter where you are, thank you to all the babies in the world for meeting us in our dreams and nesting safely in our hearts.